Other books coauthored by Mike Samuels,
with Hal Z. Bennett:

The Well Body Book
Spirit Guides: Access to Inner Worlds
Be Well
Well Body, Well Earth

By Mike Samuels and Nancy Samuels:

*Seeing With the Mind's Eye: The History,
Techniques, and Uses of Visualization*
The Well Pregnancy Book
The Well Child Book
The Well Child Coloring Book
The Well Adult
The Well Baby Book

By Mike Samuels
Healing With the Mind's Eye

HYPERTENSION

HOW TO WORK
WITH YOUR DOCTOR AND
TAKE CHARGE OF YOUR HEALTH

Mike Samuels, M.D.,
and
Nancy Samuels

SUMMIT BOOKS

New York   London   Toronto   Sydney   Tokyo   Singapore

SUMMIT BOOKS
SIMON & SCHUSTER BUILDING
ROCKEFELLER CENTER
1230 AVENUE OF THE AMERICAS
NEW YORK, NEW YORK, 10020

SUMMIT BOOKS AND COLOPHON ARE TRADEMARKS
OF SIMON & SCHUSTER INC.

DESIGNED BY IRVING PERKINS ASSOCIATES
MANUFACTURED IN THE UNITED STATES OF AMERICA

1   3   5   7   9   10   8   6   4   2

LIBRARY OF CONGRESS CATALOGING IN PUBLICATION DATA

Samuels, Mike.
Hypertension: how to work with your doctor and take charge of
your health / Mike Samuels and Nancy Samuels.
p.   cm.
1. Hypertension—Popular works.   I. Samuels, Nancy.   II. Title.
RC685.H8S254   1991
616.1'32—dc20   91-27778
CIP
ISBN: 0-671-68216-4

The ideas, procedures, and suggestions in this book are not intended as a substitute for the medical advice of a trained health professional. All matters regarding your health require medical supervision. Consult your physician before adopting the suggestions in this book, as well as about any condition that may require diagnosis or medical attention. The publishers and authors disclaim any liability arising directly or indirectly from the use of the techniques in this book.

Acknowledgments

We would like to thank Jim Silberman for supporting this series of books on taking charge of illness, Dominick Anfuso for editorial care, and Elaine Markson for being there. We would also like to thank Dr. Jerald Young for reading parts of the manuscript and giving us suggestions, Joel and Charlotte Reiter for doing pioneering work in the take control approach, and Marshall and Phyllis Klaus for inspiration in patient support. Finally, we would like to thank family and friends, in particular Rudy and Lewis, for love and support.

Acknowledgments

For Iggy Samuels

Contents

HYPERTENSION

CHAPTER ONE

Taking Charge

Taking charge of your hypertension can help you feel better and live longer. It will give you a means of lowering your blood pressure, thereby preventing the possibility of the consequences that can result from uncontrolled high blood pressure. In most instances, hypertension is a disease that is *very* responsive to treatment, but unlike some other illnesses, much of the success of the treatment is up to you. Hypertension is not a disease that has early symptoms that cause people to seek treatment. Currently, there is no way to predict who is likely to be seriously affected by the disease, so doctors recommend that everyone's blood pressure be kept at levels that are considered safe. If high blood pressure is lowered through some form of treatment, then stroke, heart failure, and kidney damage can be prevented, and the risk of heart attack can be lessened. The message of this book is simply that by your own actions, you can take charge of this disease.

First, we want to reassure you. High blood pressure can readily be controlled in virtually everyone. As long as your blood pressure is under control, there's no reason to be anxious about the health hazards associated with hypertension. Our message is to take charge of your blood pressure so you can stop worrying about it. You do not need to be frightened of having high blood pressure, but you do need to deal with the condition. Fortunately there is much that can be done for high blood pressure. First, lifestyle changes involving stress reduction, dietary adjustments, and exercise can often completely control mild hypertension or help lower the necessary dosage of drugs. Second, a

9

variety of medications, including several new ones, have made drug therapy more effective, with fewer side effects. Either type of treatment regimen requires personal action and commitment; both require a decision to *take charge of your health*. To do this, you need to clearly understand the nature of the disease, why treatment is necessary, and how the various types of treatment work. If people do not understand the value of a treatment regimen, they are less likely to sustain it for any length of time.

Why take charge?

Because hypertension is a symptomless illness, but a potentially serious risk factor, it presents a paradox. On the one hand, people with hypertension usually do not feel sick, and therefore are not very motivated to make lifestyle changes or take medication. On the other hand, some people who are diagnosed with hypertension suddenly view themselves as "sick," and constantly worry about the long-range consequences of their condition. Although both of these reactions are natural, neither is helpful over the long-term. Ignoring high blood pressure can have serious consequences, but worrying makes people feel badly and can even contribute to a rise in their blood pressure by stimulating the sympathetic nervous system. Taking charge provides a different approach and produces a different attitude. First, it treats the problem and helps to prevent future illness. Secondly, it relieves worry and replaces feelings of helplessness with feelings of control, which further helps to lower blood pressure by reducing sympathetic arousal. Taking charge not only makes people feel better, it can actually help cure the illness.

We use *taking charge* in a global sense—not only dealing specifically with a person's hypertension, but dealing with the rest of a person's life as well. In order to make effective lifestyle changes or take medication on a regular basis, people must create a positive attitude toward managing their condition. This process is enhanced when people act to improve other areas of their life. It is important to keep in perspective the fact that hypertension is only one facet of a person's life. More broadly, people's attitude or world view affects the way they deal with their illness. When people feel a sense of control over their lives, they are more likely to believe that their own actions can affect their destiny. If people have a sense of fulfillment, personally and spiritually, they are more likely to act in a way that will have a positive effect on their life. Optimally, taking charge will improve your life in ways that go far beyond simply dealing with your hypertension. We hope that the process of taking charge of your high blood pressure will result in a greater sense of personal fulfillment and a greater sense of control over the rest of your life.

Although people with hypertension need to be under a doctor's care, they *themselves* will be largely responsible for how well their medical treatment works. Once hypertension has been diagnosed, follow-up visits to the doctor are generally brief: blood pressure is checked, lab tests may be done, and therapy is discussed. But the real treatment takes place in the weeks and months between visits. It is during this time that a person actually undertakes those changes that will bring his or her blood pressure down to an acceptable level. Studies have shown that the major reason for inadequate control of hypertension—and the diseases that it can cause—is the fact that over a long period of time many people with high blood pressure do not maintain healthy lifestyle changes and/or continue to take their medication regularly. Other studies have shown that educational programs and planned strategies for dealing with hypertension significantly increase blood pressure control, as well as health and longevity.

The basic goal of this book is to help people create a comprehensive program that is tailored for them. Individualized programs that people are actively involved in developing for themselves are the ones most likely to be successful over a long period of time. Every person is unique, and every person reacts differently to the various aspects of a comprehensive program. Some people are very interested in and highly motivated to work on stress reduction, some on nutritional change, and some on exercise. Some people readily accept the idea of medication, others are very motivated to work at lifestyle changes in an effort to stay off anti-hypertensive drugs or lower their dosages. Every person who is on some form of medication for high blood pressure needs to work with their doctor to find the medication and dosage that will be the most effective for them and have the least side effects. When people actively work with their doctor to tailor their own program, they are more likely to carry it out and be successful in achieving long-term control over their blood pressure.

Body, mind, and spirit

It has long been known that blood pressure is affected by stress and emotions. The classic example of this effect is that people's blood pressure frequently goes up when it is taken in a doctor's office. This phenomenon is so well-known that it is referred to as "white-coat hypertension." Doctors believe it is due to the fact that patients are often anxious when they are going to be examined by a doctor. Recent research has led doctors to think that for many people stress may play a *causal* role in the early stages of hypertension. When people perceive themselves as being under stress, their sympathetic nervous system is alerted. Messages from the sympathetic nervous system cause the heart to pump harder and faster, which in turn makes blood pressure rise. This phenomenon is part of a natural adaptation that prepares our bodies for escape from danger. Some experts think that if this type of arousal occurs often enough over a period of years, the walls of the blood vessels eventually become thickened. As a result, blood pressure remains continuously elevated because it is harder for the heart to push the blood against the increased resistance in the walls. The most recent studies have shown that the sympathetic nervous system raises blood pressure by a very complex mechanism that involves the kidneys' retaining salt and water to regulate the fluid level in the body.

Relaxation and stress reduction have long been known to quiet the sympathetic nervous system and lower blood pressure. It is also known that certain attitudes, such as a sense of control, can reduce a person's perception of being under stress. Furthermore, feelings of fulfillment and spiritual connectedness help people cope with stress. Thus the whole concept of taking charge of one's life may lessen or prevent hypertension in a more global sense, above and beyond the ways in which specific lifestyle changes and drugs work to lower blood pressure. It's as if the *take charge* model constitutes a life change in and of itself. Taking charge is transformative, it causes you to evaluate your whole life in a new way. Determining which among various alternatives will be best for your health naturally leads to considering what in your life would be most beneficial or fulfilling for you. This kind of thinking increases your sense of control, your sense of involvement, and your perception of being able to meet the challenges in your life. Such a change in consciousness or attitude lessens feelings of helplessness and stress, and helps to lower blood pressure by itself.

The *take charge* program

The *take charge* program is divided into four parts. The first step is *deciding to take charge of your hypertension*. Such a decision is the initial step in any action or plan that a person undertakes. What's necessary in order to make the decision is knowledge—the knowledge that you have high blood pressure (or are at risk of developing it), the knowledge that hypertension generally does not produce symptoms that alert you to its existence, and the knowledge that in a definite percentage of people hypertension will eventually result in serious illness if it is allowed to go untreated. Armed with this knowledge, people will better understand their condition and be able to set realistic goals for lowering their blood pressure so as to optimize their health.

The second step in a *take charge* program involves *taking action*. To decide on a course of action, you need to know what lifestyle changes specifically lower blood pressure, which may be all that's necessary to achieve control. You also need to know that if your blood pressure cannot be reduced by lifestyle changes alone, drugs will be necessary in addition for effective control. The particular drug-and-lifestyle regimen should be worked out in conjunction with your doctor in such a way as to best enhance the quality of your life.

The third step in the program is *taking control of your treatment*. This involves monitoring your blood pressure (at home or in the doctor's office) and evaluating the effectiveness of your treatment regime. This process takes place over a period of months, and generally will involve some modifications in your lifestyle and perhaps in your drug therapy.

The fourth step in the *take charge* program, which applies to any chronic illness, is *maintaining optimal treatment over a long period of time*. This means sticking to the program you've developed with

TAKING CHARGE OF YOUR HYPERTENSION

Step 1. Decide to take charge.
High blood pressure does not produce symptoms, but can result in serious illness if left untreated.

Step 2. Take action.
Work out optimum lifestyle changes, and if necessary, drug therapy, in conjunction with your doctor.

Step 3. Take control of your treatment.
Monitor blood pressure regularly, at home or in the doctor's office, and evaluate the effectiveness of your treatment regimen.

Step 4. Continue to maintain optimum control.
Make lifestyle changes and drug modifications as necessary in order to feel your best and keep blood pressure in optimum control.

your doctor, maintaining your motivation, and adapting to changes in your own condition and new knowledge and drugs used to treat hypertension.

How to use this book

Hypertension: How to Work with Your Doctor and Take Charge of Your Health consists of eight chapters, the goal of which is to give you the knowledge and skill to implement the *take charge* program. Chapter Two explains what hypertension is and why it needs to be treated. Chapters Three, Four, and Five deal with lifestyle changes, or what doctors refer to as "nonpharmacological treatment." Chapter Three discusses the complex relationship between blood pressure and the mind, and describes how stress, attitude, relaxation, imagery, and support affect blood pressure. Chapter Four deals with the ways in which dietary factors such as weight reduction, sodium, alcohol, and smoking affect blood pressure. Chapter Five examines the value of aerobic exercise in relation to hypertension. Chapter Six gives a concise explanation of how the different blood pressure medications work, and what their common side effects are. Chapter Seven deals with the complex relationship between hypertension, antihypertensive medications, and sexual function. Finally, the last chapter deals with incorporating all the knowledge you have gleaned into an effective personal program.

As we've said, a diagnosis of hypertension should be a cause for concern but not worry since long-range problems are preventable as long as high blood pressure is brought under control. Working in conjunction with your doctor, you can make effective lifestyle changes, and, if necessary, take medication that has minimal side effects. We believe that taking charge will do more for you than control your hypertension. The program will give you the opportunity and the attitude necessary to take charge of other aspects of your life, enhancing it and making it more fulfilling. No one wants to have an illness, but people often find, to their surprise, that an illness can bring positive as well as negative changes. An illness forces people to refocus, to evaluate what is truly important in their life, to set up priorities, and to spend time in activities that they truly enjoy. It makes people focus on the here and now, and value those things that are often taken for granted—the joy of the natural world, the simple pleasures of a day, and interactions with people they love.

CHAPTER TWO

What Is Hypertension?

In order to deal effectively with hypertension, people need a clear understanding of what the disease is and what treatment can accomplish. For people to become involved in their own care, they have to understand the physiology of the disease and why doctors feel that treatment is so important. When people understand the disease and are aware of the advantages of treatment, they can make the decision to control their blood pressure. This is the first step in the *take charge* program.

Hypertension is one of the most common of all illnesses. Doctors estimate that 60 million Americans, some 15 to 20% of the population, have high blood pressure. Many more are at risk because of family history or other factors. So if you have hypertension, you are certainly not alone. Even though almost all of the people with high blood pressure have *no* symptoms, many well-designed studies show that for some of them, long-term untreated hypertension will lead to congestive heart failure, strokes, kidney failure, and heart attacks. With adequate treatment, most of these problems can be prevented. In fact, since 1972 the number of deaths from strokes has been cut in half due to the fact that more people with high blood pressure are diagnosed early and maintain adequate treatment over a long period of time. Still, there are many people who do not realize that they have high blood pressure, and a quarter to a half of those who are diagnosed eventually discontinue treatment. Studies indicate that one of the major reasons people stop treatment is that they are not involved in their own care.

Hypertension consists of persistent elevated pressure in the arteries, and the consequences of that rise. Stated in this way, it sounds simple, but in fact, the disease is quite complex and not completely understood. Many factors affect arterial pressure. Blood pressure normally varies with time of day, activity level, and emotional state. When doctors speak of a person's blood pressure, they base it on several readings taken at rest, usually in their office. Such a figure is considered average because blood pressure always goes up with exertion or stress, and goes down during sleep.

Levels of hypertension that require treatment

One of the problems in defining what constitutes high blood pressure is the fact that within a given population people naturally range from relatively low to relatively high values, with most people having values somewhere in the middle. Put in graph form, the values form a bell-shaped curve. Both medical data and insurance studies show that medical problems increase as blood pressure increases, starting with the lowest figures. For doctors, the problem has been to ascertain at what values there are sufficient problems to label blood pressure as too high and to institute some kind of treatment. There is no firm dividing line below which there is no incidence of stroke, kidney disease, or heart disease. Nor does everyone above a certain level develop these problems. Rather, as blood pressure increases, so does the *probability* of experiencing a stroke, kidney disease, or heart disease. It's important to reiterate that hypertension is a *risk factor* for these illnesses; it is not a one-to-one, cause-and-effect situation. In fact, 85% of people with *significant* hypertension are at no greater risk of these diseases than the average person, and 99% of people with *mild* hypertension are at no greater risk. It is the small subgroup of hypertensives that is at much greater than average risk who are really helped by treatment.

Doctors treat everyone with significant high blood pressure because they still cannot precisely identify who is at great risk. In general, the higher a person's blood pressure readings, the higher the risk. Other factors thought to help identify those people who will most benefit from treatment are a family history of high blood pressure, a personal history of heart disease, a high cholesterol level, and/or kidney disease.

RISK FACTORS FOR HEART DISEASE

Smoking

High blood pressure

High cholesterol level

Lack of exercise

High stress

High salt intake

Heavy drinking

Family history of heart disease

Obesity

Male gender

SELF-CARE FOR HIGH BLOOD PRESSURE

1. Eat a low-salt, low-cholesterol diet.
2. Maintain a reasonable weight.
3. Do aerobic exercise 3–5 times a week.
4. Learn ways to effectively cope with stress.
5. Stop smoking.
6. Meditate or do relaxation exercises daily.
7 Motivate lifestyle changes by learning about the dangers of high blood pressure.
8. Take medication regularly if prescribed by a doctor.

In 1984 the Joint National Committee on Detection, Evaluation, and Treatment of High Blood Pressure agreed on the blood pressure values at which they felt treatment was necessary. Basically, they recommended that blood pressure above 140/90 be considered as hypertension and be addressed with some form of treatment.

The physiology of high blood pressure

In order to develop a better understanding of hypertension, it is important to learn about those factors—mechanical, physical, and emotional—that affect blood pressure. Blood pressure is simply the force that the blood exerts against the walls of the arteries. The blood in the arteries is under pressure because the arteries and veins essentially form a closed system containing sufficient blood to cause pressure on the walls even when the heart is not pumping. This "resting" pressure is the lower of the two values in a blood pressure reading. It is called the *diastolic pressure*. When the heart beats, it pumps the blood through the system under increased pressure. This "pumping" pressure is the upper value in a blood pressure reading, and it is called the *systolic pressure*.

Without some pressure in the system, the heart would not be able to pump the blood up to the brain or out to the extremities. Pressure is necessary in order to make the blood flow, or move, against gravity and against the resistance of the arterial walls. The resistance is caused by friction, and it increases with the length of the artery and decreases as the artery gets wider. In mathematical terms, the amount of blood flow is proportional to the fourth power of the diameter. This means that if the diameter increases from 1 to 2 millimeters, the flow increases 16 times, and if the diameter increases from 1 to 4 millimeters, the flow increases 256 times. As you can see, very slight changes in blood vessel width have tremendous effects on blood flow. Thus, generally, if a blood vessel contracts even slightly, the pressure on the artery walls goes up measurably since the same amount of blood is being pumped through the artery. What's of greater consequence is that if the arteries don't relax and expand when stress is reduced, blood pressure remains higher than it should be.

Blood pressure depends on two basic factors: the resistance of the small arteries and the pumping of the heart. The amount the heart pumps, which is referred to as *cardiac output*, is highly variable. It depends on both how fast the heart beats and how much blood it pumps out with each beat, that is, how strongly it beats. The total amount of fluid in the circulatory system also affects cardiac output: the more blood in the system, the greater the pressure. Cardiac output varies from an average of 5 liters per minute at rest, to an average of 20 to 30 liters per minute during heavy exercise. The resistance of the small arteries, which is called *peripheral resistance,* is related to their diameter, which varies according to how much the muscles in the walls of the arteries contract. Blood pressure can then be expressed in a simple formula:

$$\text{blood pressure} = \text{cardiac output} \times \text{peripheral resistance}$$

Thus when the heart beats faster or harder, blood pressure goes up; likewise, when the arteries contract or become more resistant to expanding, blood pressure goes up.

The remarkable thing about the circulatory system is that it is able to adapt to widely varying conditions, and generally maintain blood pressure within a safe range. Blood pressure is the lowest when the body is at rest, lying down. If a person sits up or moves, the body is able to respond and keep a fairly stable pressure. When a person exercises, blood pressure must increase in order to circulate more blood, and thus more oxygen, to the skeletal muscles. The body has exquisite mechanisms to maintain blood pressure at a level sufficient to supply all the cells with enough oxygen and food, but low enough to ensure that no damage is done to the heart, blood vessels or kidneys. If any of these mechanisms fails to operate properly, or if the arteries become hardened and less elastic, then the average blood pressure increases and remains elevated.

How the body regulates blood pressure

One of the most important mechanisms affecting blood pressure levels is the *autonomic nervous system,* the part of the nervous system that is responsible for those functions such as breathing that the body carries on automatically. The *sympathetic* branch of the autonomic nervous system facilitates rapid variations in blood pressure necessitated by changes in posture and temperature, or by dangerous situations that require quick action. The sympathetic nervous system has both incoming nerves that bring messages to the brain and outgoing nerves that cause changes in other parts of the body. Special receptors in the carotid arteries of the neck and in the aortic arch, the largest artery emerging from the heart, continuously monitor blood pressure. When blood pressure drops, these receptors signal the *vasomotor center* in the brain stem, which in turn stimulates the sympathetic nervous system. Sympathetic nerves leading to the heart and blood vessels do not stimulate muscle tissue directly, rather they release a chemical, *norepineph-rine*, which promotes the uptake of calcium which is necessary in order for muscle tissue to contract. In the heart, norepinephrine acts on *beta receptors* which are on the surface of the muscle tissue, causing an increase in both the strength and rate of the heartbeat. In the *arterioles*, the network of small arteries throughout the body, norepinephrine is taken up by *alpha receptors*, causing the muscle layer in the arterioles to contract, increasing resistance and causing blood pressure to go up. Thus the sympathetic nervous system affects both factors in the blood pressure equation—cardiac output and peripheral resistance.

When stimulated, the sympathetic nervous system causes the muscles in arterial walls to contract and the heart to beat faster and harder, a combination of events which raises blood pressure instantly. For example, when people stand up, gravity exerts a downward force on the blood. This would leave the brain and heart with too little blood were it not for the sympathetic receptors in the carotid arteries which alert the brain to raise blood pressure instantly.

The body also has mechanisms that work to lower blood pressure. Basically, blood pressure is lowered by a *decrease* in sympathetic nervous system activity. Thus if the body is not being aroused, it returns to a resting state that is more relaxed. This decrease in arousal is facilitated by the *parasympathetic* branch of the autonomic nervous system. The parasympathetic nerve leading to the heart is called the *vagus*. When stimulated, its fibers release a chemical called *acetylcho-line*, which causes the heart to beat more slowly and with less force. At any given moment, both the heart's rate and output are controlled by a combination of parasympathetic and sympathetic activity.

A number of researchers now believe that the autonomic nervous system plays an important role in the initiation of high blood pressure, and its continuation. Research has shown that the majority of people who have just developed hypertension have abnormal sympathetic and parasympathetic control mechanisms as shown by a slightly elevated heart rate, above average cardiac output, and higher than average blood levels of norepinephrine. In general, these people also show a greater than average blood pressure rise in response to psychological stress. Conversely, their blood pressure drops to a greater degree in response to sleep and relaxation. The fact that blood pressure rises in response to stress is thought to explain why blood pressure values tend to be higher in stressful cultures and societies undergoing social change.

The second major mechanism that mediates blood pressure involves the kidneys. The kidneys secrete an enzyme called *renin,* which causes blood pressure to rise. Increased amounts of this enzyme are normally released when the sympathetic nervous system is aroused, when the amount of sodium is low in the kidneys, or when blood pressure in the kidneys falls due to postural changes or even bleeding. When renin enters the bloodstream, it breaks down a common protein, producing *angiotensin* I. In the lungs, angiotensin I encounters *angiotensin converting enzyme (ACE)* which is always present in high amounts. ACE converts angiotensin I to *angiotensin* II, a substance which causes an immediate and powerful clamping down of the arterioles, directly raising the blood pressure. Angiotensin II also causes the kidneys to retain salt, which increases blood pressure indirectly and more gradually by increasing the body's fluid volume. The renin system is considered a major long-term regulator of blood pressure and salt balance.

The third major mechanism which affects blood pressure maintenance is the ability of the kidneys to handle salt, or, more precisely, the sodium in salt. By retaining or excreting water and sodium, the kidneys regulate the body's volume of blood, which in turn affects blood pressure. The higher the body's blood volume, the harder the heart has to pump, both because there is more blood to circulate and because there is more resistance in the arteries. Thus blood pressure rises. As blood pressure increases, the body naturally tends to excrete more urine in order to reduce blood volume. A flaw in the way the kidneys handle sodium and water is probably an important factor in many cases of high blood pressure. The majority of people with hypertension have low renin levels and they exhibit a diminished capacity to excrete sodium when their blood pressure goes up in response to increased fluid levels.

To recap, blood pressure is the result of cardiac output (flow) multiplied by peripheral resistance. Both flow and resistance are increased by sympathetic nervous system arousal. In addition, resistance goes up when the kidneys' renin system causes the arterioles to clamp down.

And both blood flow and resistance go up when the kidneys retain salt and water, thereby increasing the blood volume.

Categories of hypertension

As we've said, high blood pressure is not simply defined as a fixed value, but rather the level at which, in light of other predisposing factors, the risk of long-range medical problems becomes great enough to warrant treatment. The present standard is 140/90, but the Joint National Committee designates several subgroups. In terms of *diastolic,* or resting, blood pressure, anything below 85 is considered normal. Between 85 and 89 is considered "high normal." Generally nothing is done for people in this range other than rechecking blood pressure periodically. A figure of 90–104 diastolic is considered *mild hypertension.* This category includes most of the people who have high blood pressure. From 105 to 114 is considered *moderate hypertension.* Above 115 is classified as *severe hypertension.* "Mild" does not mean that the level is unimportant, rather, it simply classifies the diastolic level in relation to even higher levels. Studies have definitely shown that even mild hypertension should receive some form of treatment—either lifestyle change or drugs.

WHAT IS HIGH BLOOD PRESSURE?

Blood pressure (in mmHg)	Category
Diastolic blood pressure	
Under 85	Normal blood pressure
85–89	High-normal blood pressure
90–104	Mild hypertension
105–114	Moderate hypertension
Over 115	Severe hypertension
Systolic blood pressure (*with diastolic under 90*)	
Under 140	Normal blood pressure
140–159	Borderline systolic hypertension
Above 160	Isolated systolic hypertension

Another type of hypertension is called *isolated systolic hypertension*. In this condition, the diastolic blood pressure is normal, that is, below 90, but the systolic blood pressure is elevated. A systolic pressure over 160 is defined as *isolated systolic hypertension,* while a value of 140–159 is considered *borderline isolated systolic hypertension.* Isolated systolic hypertension is most common in people over 55. When it occurs in younger people, it often is a predictor for later diastolic hypertension. The basic goal of all hypertension treatment is to reduce blood pressure to 140/90 or lower, or below 160 in isolated systolic hypertension. In the case of mild hypertension, the decision on how to treat the problem varies depending on a person's other risk factors.

The causes of high blood pressure

The cause or causes of most cases of hypertension are not currently known. In fact, in the great majority of patients (90–95%), high blood pressure does not have a single, definable cause. This type of hypertension is referred to as *essential* or *primary hypertension*. Most doctors believe that this type represents a variety of physiological conditions which raise cardiac output, increase peripheral resistance, and/or affect sodium balance. In different people one of these mechanisms may be more important than the others, thus treatment differs accordingly. The other 5% of hypertension cases are classed as *secondary hypertension*. The causes of secondary hypertension can be diagnosed, and often can be treated. Causes include use of oral contraceptives; various types of kidney disease, including narrowing of the arteries to the kidneys; toxemia in pregnancy; and more rarely, thyroid conditions and adrenal tumors.

Although the underlying causes of primary hypertension are generally not known, there are certain factors that predispose people to high blood pressure. One that has long been recognized is *genetics*. Over three-quarters of the people with high blood pressure have a family history of the disease. However, the problem is not a simple, one-gene condition that is passed directly from parent to child.

Age is a factor in some societies. In most cultures, blood pressure increases with age, but there are some cultures in which it does not. Although hypertension is usually picked up during middle age, it is thought to begin during young adulthood. At that point, blood pressure values are not generally in the disease range, probably because the body is still able to adjust sufficiently to keep the blood pressure within normal limits. However, as people grow older, several changes may occur. First, the body's pressure receptors in the blood vessels and the kidneys may be reset so that the body does not respond as appropriately to increases in blood pressure. Second, the blood vessels may become thickened and less elastic, and may develop cholesterol plaques.

Sodium intake is another factor in the development of hypertension. It has long been noted that societies which consume high amounts of salt have a greater percentage of people with hypertension. Within a given culture, those people who consume high amounts of salt are more likely to develop hypertension, as are people who emigrate from a low-salt to a high-salt culture.

Another established risk factor for hypertension is *obesity*. People who are overweight are more likely to have high blood pressure at any given age. This is most likely due to the increase in blood volume experienced by people as they put on weight. Interestingly, studies show that increased eating also causes an increase in sympathetic nervous system activity.

Why hypertension should be treated
High blood pressure should be treated simply because it is a significant risk factor for strokes, heart attacks, and kidney disease—serious conditions which can cause premature disability and death. As we've said, not everyone with untreated hypertension will develop one of these conditions, only a small minority will. But currently there is no way to determine which people are truly at risk. With effective treatment to lower blood pressure, the risk of these conditions can be greatly lowered for all people who have hypertension.

A number of large, well-designed studies have shown the average age of onset for hypertension to be in the early 30s. Without treatment for moderate-to-severe hypertension, men in these studies were found to have a mean survival of 20 years, whereas the normal survival was 40 years. Thus for men who developed mild hypertension in their 30s,

**HYPERTENSION AND MORTALITY:
INCREASED MORTALITY DUE TO ELEVATED DIASTOLIC BLOOD
PRESSURE AS COMPARED WITH OVERALL MORTALITY RATES**

Diastolic blood in mmHg	64–84	84–88	89–93	94–103
*Deaths	95	100	116	151

* Actual to expected deaths. Expected = 100.

their mean survival was many years less than normal. Again, most of the men in these studies did not develop strokes, kidney disease, or heart disease, but enough did, and did so at an early age, to reduce the overall life expectancy of the untreated hypertensive group by many years. Large, well-designed studies have also shown that with adequate treatment, hypertensives could largely prevent these complications. The Veterans Administration Cooperative Study on Hypertension showed a reduction of serious illness from 55% to 18% with adequate treatment.

The relationship between hypertension and complications such as stroke, kidney disease, and heart disease

The most common illness developed by people with hypertension is actually *coronary artery disease*. It is usually caused by the development of fibro-fatty plaques that narrow the major arteries, including the arteries of the heart. This process, which is called *atherosclerosis*, is the major cause of heart attacks and angina, and is also the cause of

YEARS OF LIFE LOST DUE TO HIGH BLOOD PRESSURE

BLOOD PRESSURE LEVELS	MEN		WOMEN	
	35	55	35	55
130/90	4 yrs.	1 yr.	2 yrs.	1 yr.
140/95	9	4	5	3
150/100	17	6	9	4

one type of stroke. Studies show that a high fat diet, high serum cholesterol levels, cigarette smoking, and lack of exercise, as well as high blood pressure are all risk factors for atherosclerosis.

The role that hypertension plays in the development of atherosclerosis is thought to be largely mechanical. When blood pressure is high, the blood pushes against the artery walls with much greater than normal force, abrading the lining. In damaged areas, the cells lining the arteries begin to proliferate. In some cases this process continues past the point of healing the abrasion, and particles of fat may be incorporated into the wall, building up a fatty plaque. Controlling blood pressure will help to alleviate, but will not stop the process of atherosclerosis, unless other risk factors for heart disease are also reduced, most importantly cholesterol levels.

Strokes are caused by two different physiological mechanisms. One, atherosclerotic blockage of the arteries leading to the brain, causes 70% of all strokes. It occurs when arteries become too constricted to allow sufficient blood to get to the brain. To reduce the likelihood of this condition, other risk factors must be controlled in addition to blood pressure. The other 30% of strokes are caused by *microaneurysms,* tiny weaknesses in the small arteries of the brain which balloon out and burst. This type of stroke is usually related to hypertension, and is preventable only if blood pressure is controlled.

Kidney disease is not a common complication of mild or moderate high blood pressure. It occurs in a small percentage of patients, usually ones with severe, uncontrolled hypertension. In this situation the muscle fibers in the walls of the tiny arteries in the kidneys actually tear, allowing blood to seep into the arterial wall, which eventually shuts down the blood vessels and causes damage to nearby tissues. Eventually, if enough tissue is damaged, kidney function can be impaired.

Controversies in hypertension treatment

Currently, there are two basic controversies about the treatment of hypertension. First, is there a single level of blood pressure above which treatment should be started in everyone? Second, can the risk of atherosclerotic heart disease be significantly reduced by treatment of hypertension, and if so, what type of treatment will be most effective from this standpoint?

Studies show that for all levels of hypertension, including mild high blood pressure, treatment reduces complications. However, as the risk of complications decreases for mild hypertension, the long-range value of treatment becomes more questionable. Mild hypertensives are at much less risk of stroke and kidney disease, and other risk factors are more important than their hypertension in terms of heart disease. In fact, some trials have even shown that 50% of patients with mild high blood pressure not only achieve normal blood pressure without any therapy, they have fewer medical problems, such as heart attacks, than people with similar blood pressure levels who are put on some form of drug therapy. For pressures above 100 diastolic, however, doctors do not question the fact that the value of drug treatment in terms of decreased complications is greater than any problems associated with drug side effects.

In treating people with pressures under 100 diastolic, there are several approaches that address the controversy. The doctor may prescribe lifestyle changes instead of drugs. Such changes not only eliminate potential side effects of medication, they address other heart disease risk factors as well, including stress, high cholesterol, alcohol, and lack of exercise. Moreover, doctors often deal with people who have mild hypertension on an individual basis, trying to identify those who are at higher risk for stroke or heart attack, and reserving drug therapy for them.

The second controversy, whether treatment of hypertension lowers the risk of heart attack, is harder to resolve. Research has shown that treatment does reduce the risk of cardiovascular complications in people with blood pressure levels over 100 diastolic. But many studies have shown little effect on the incidence of heart disease in people with under 100 diastolic, although some research has shown a small positive effect. Interestingly, several studies show a slight, but definite, cardio-protective effect from the use of beta-blocker drugs. On the other hand, it has been found that some drugs, such as diuretics, raise blood lipid and cholesterol levels. In terms of heart attack, this response may outweigh the beneficial effects of lowering blood pressure. Thus doctors must take a person's heart disease risk factors and history into consideration when choosing a course of therapy for hypertension.

How blood pressure is measured

Blood pressure is measured with a *sphygmomanometer,* a simple device that consists of an inflatable balloon inside a nylon sleeve, or cuff, which is loosely secured around the upper arm with a Velcro fastening. The cuff is inflated with a small hand pump to put pressure on the arteries of the upper arm. The pump is also connected to a column of mercury in a glass tube, or to a pressure gauge. Blood pressure is measured in millimeters of mercury (mmHg) because this was standard in the earliest devices, and it is still found in the cuffs used by many doctors because this type of gauge gives the most accurate reading. With the older type of gauge, the person taking the blood pressure puts the bell of a stethoscope beneath the cuff in order to hear the sound of the blood hitting the artery wall. The newer style of cuff, which measures the sound of the blood electronically, is not as accurate as the mercury sphygmomanometer, or mechanical gauge.

When a cuff is sufficiently inflated, it functions like a tourniquet, and the pressure exerted collapses the artery wall and temporarily shuts off blood flow. At this point the pressure in the cuff is higher than the pressure in the artery. The person taking the blood pressure then slowly lets the air out of the cuff, listening intently with the stethoscope for the first sound of blood again flowing through the artery. As the pressure in the cuff becomes equal to the pressure in the artery, the artery reopens and blood flows through, making a sound as it hits the compressed wall of the artery. The person hears a tapping noise as a wave of blood from each beat of the heart hits the narrowed wall. These sounds, which were first discovered in 1905, are referred to as *Korotkov sounds.* The sound that is first heard as the cuff is deflated is called *phase one* of the Korotkov sounds. It represents the pressure produced when the heart pumps, and is known as the *systolic blood pressure.*

As air continues to be let out of the cuff, sounds continue to be heard until the pressure in the cuff drops below the level at which the artery is compressed. At this point, blood flows easily through the vessel and there is no noise of blood hitting the walls. This represents *phase five*

HOW TO TAKE YOUR OWN BLOOD PRESSURE

Step 1. Get your stethoscope and blood pressure cuff and sit where you will be able to rest your forearm comfortably about on a level with your heart.

Step 2. Sit quietly for five minutes. If you are nervous, let yourself relax.

Step 3. Arrange clothing so the area above your elbow is bare. Wrap cuff snugly around your upper arm; secure with the Velcro lock or D-ring. Make sure that the mark or the tubes coming out of the cuff are approximately in line with the artery in the crook of your arm. Put the earpieces of the stethoscope in your ears, and put the bell over the brachial artery, in the top center of your forearm, directly below the cuff.

Step 4. Close the control knob on the bulb, then squeeze the bulb until the number on the pressure gauge is at least 20 points above your usual systolic blood pressure. Release the control knob slightly until the pressure gauge starts to drop. As the pressure drops, listen for the sounds to appear. Note the number on the gauge when the first sound appears. This is the systolic blood pressure. Continue to let the pressure drop, and listen for all sound to disappear. Again note the number. This is the diastolic blood pressure. Let the pressure drop all the way to 0, wait a minute or so, then repeat the procedure again. If the second reading is lower, repeat the procedure until the values match.

of the Korotkov sounds, and is called the *diastolic blood pressure.* Diastolic pressure coincides with the resting phase between heartbeats when the heart is refilling. It represents the maintenance level of pressure within the circulatory system. Blood pressure is recorded as two numbers: the systolic over the diastolic. For example, 140/90 mmHg means the systolic, or pumping, pressure is 140, while the diastolic, or resting, pressure is 90. Historically, the diastolic blood pressure has been the one used in research studies and has been considered to be the more significant in predicting the likelihood of stroke, kidney disease, and heart disease. In recent years, however, studies have shown that systolic blood pressure is also important, perhaps even more important than the diastolic. Now both values are looked at carefully by doctors.

Diagnosing hypertension

A diagnosis of high blood pressure, or hypertension, is made on the basis of a number of blood pressure readings. Because it is now known that blood pressure varies with many factors such as stress and exertion, readings are generally taken on several occasions over a period of time. This is especially important if blood pressure is only mildly elevated. In recent years doctors have come to recognize a phenomenon they call "white-coat hypertension." They have found that both diastolic and systolic readings can be as much as 30 points higher in the doctor's office than at home. Interestingly, pressures are generally highest when taken by doctors, and somewhat lower when taken by nurses. These results graphically reflect the role that anxiety, stress, and sympathetic arousal play in the regulation of blood pressure. Studies have shown that 20–30% of people with mild hypertension (90–104 diastolic) show high pressures in the office, but not at other times. Doctors do not consider this to be true hypertension.

A diagnosis of hypertension is based on the average of repeated high values that remain elevated regardless of when or where they are taken. Most doctors base a diagnosis on two or three measurements taken on two or three separate occasions. In the case of people with mild hypertension or people who seem to be very anxious in the office, the doctor may demonstrate how to use a cuff, and then have them check their blood pressure at home at regular intervals. Sometimes the doctor will even have patients get used to taking their own blood pressure before they begin recording values. Often the values drop down to a lower level as people become more used to taking their blood pressure.

In order for blood pressure readings to be accurate, it is suggested that people follow certain guidelines:

1) Rest quietly for five minutes before taking your blood pressure.

2) Sit with your arm at chest height.

3) Be sure the cuff is the right size—the balloon inside the sleeve should encircle at least two-thirds of the upper arm. (People who have very large biceps or who are overweight may need a larger-size cuff.)

4) Two or more readings should be taken at each sitting, and the results should be averaged. If the figures are very divergent, a third reading should be taken.

5) Do not smoke or drink any caffeinated beverage within 30 minutes of taking your blood pressure (both cause a temporary elevation of blood pressure).

6) For the purposes of record keeping, do not take your blood pressure only when you *fear* it is high; in addition, take it on a regular basis when you are relaxed and at rest.

The initial hypertension workup

Before recommending a treatment plan for hypertension, the doctor will do a thorough evaluation of the patient that includes a history, a complete physical, diagnostic tests, and lab work. First, the doctor will want to determine that the person's average blood pressure actually is above the recommended level. In addition, the doctor will rule out other conditions that might be the cause of secondary hypertension, determine whether hypertension has already affected any organs, and verify any other risk factors in the person's background or lifestyle. Generally, the initial workup requires several office visits. Mild hypertension often requires more visits than moderate or severe hypertension in order to determine if the person's blood pressure is truly elevated.

The history. In taking a history, the doctor is interested in whether the patient has had heart disease, kidney disease, diabetes, or signs of a stroke. The doctor will want to know if the person has previously been diagnosed with high blood pressure, what medication was given (if any), and if the medication had any side effects. The doctor will ask if there is any family history of high blood pressure, stroke, and/or heart disease. Finally, the doctor will assess lifestyle factors such as nutrition, salt intake, alcohol consumption, previous cholesterol levels, smoking, exercise, emotional stress, and fulfillment. The doctor will also want to know of any drugs the person has taken recently, including oral contraceptives, steroids, nonsteroidal anti-inflammatory agents, cold remedies (specifically decongestants), appetite suppressants, and antidepressants.

The doctor will also inquire about symptoms in organs that can be affected by hypertension. Most people with mild or moderate high blood pressure will not have experienced such symptoms, but individuals with very high blood pressure may have. These symptoms include shortness of breath, palpitations (rapid heart beat), blurred vision, and frequent urination. Somewhat surprisingly, headaches and dizziness are not usually symptoms of hypertension, and they are no more frequent in people with high blood pressure than in individuals whose blood pressure is normal. Underlying medical conditions can produce secondary hypertension, but it is unusual, accounting for only 5–10% of all cases. These conditions have a variety of seemingly unrelated symptoms which the doctor will inquire about in order to rule out the possibility of any of these causes. Symptoms include excessive perspiration, weight loss, tremor, and muscle weakness.

The physical exam. For a person with mild or moderate high blood pressure, the physical exam will not reveal anything out of the ordinary, and will show the person to be basically healthy. In a hypertension workup, the physical is designed to do three things. First, it verifies the blood pressure. Second, it establishes that elevated blood pressure has not harmed any susceptible organs. Third, it helps to rule out secondary causes of hypertension. For this reason, parts of the exam may not seem related to blood pressure at all. During the exam, blood pressure readings are generally taken in both arms; often they are taken both sitting down and standing up. Frequently, a blood pressure reading is repeated after a period of time has elapsed.

As part of the physical, the doctor will examine the retinas of the eyes with a funduscope. Only the blood vessels in the eyes can readily be seen, and they give the doctor an indication of whether or not hypertension has affected the blood vessels. The doctor also feels or listens to the carotid arteries of the neck and checks to see if the thyroid gland is enlarged. Then the doctor listens to the heart, checking its size, rate, and the character of the heart sounds. These findings give the doctor an indication of whether the heart has had to do extra work as a result of elevated blood pressure. The doctor checks the abdomen, feeling the kidneys and listening for blood sounds in the renal arteries and the abdominal aorta, which supplies blood to the lower part of the body. The doctor will also check the pulses in both arms and legs. All this gives a more complete indication of the condition of the blood vessels throughout the body. Finally, the doctor will do a brief neurological exam, which establishes that the head and neck are receiving adequate blood flow. Again, in examining most people, particularly those with mild or moderate hypertension, the doctor is not likely to find anything of concern on the physical exam.

Lab tests. Lab tests will be done to verify the findings of the physical, and to add further information to the picture the doctor is developing. Blood will be drawn to measure hemoglobin (which reflects the number of red blood cells); potassium and calcium; creatine and blood urea nitrogen; triglycerides and cholesterol, including HDLs (high-density lipoproteins which pick up cholesterol and return it to the liver) and LDLs (low-density lipoproteins which transport cholesterol to the cells); a fasting blood sugar (blood drawn after not eating overnight); uric acid, and possibly plasma renin. These tests give information about kidney function, heart disease risk factors, and whether the person might have diabetes or gout. They also help to rule out secondary causes of hypertension. The plasma renin test, which is sometimes done, helps to evaluate the role renin plays in causing the person's hypertension, and may be important in determining what drug therapy will be most effective.

Diagnostic tests. The general workup for hypertension does not include any uncomfortable or invasive tests. A *chest x-ray* and an *electrocardiogram (ECG)* are usually done. Both indicate whether or not the heart has become enlarged in response to pumping against greater than average resistance. The ECG can also show signs of other types of heart disease. If the person has very high blood pressure readings or other significant risk factors for heart disease, the doctor may do an *echocardiogram,* a test that is more accurate in establishing whether the heart is enlarged. Additional lab tests will be done if there is a question of secondary hypertension.

By the end of the workup, the doctor will have determined if the patient actually has high blood pressure; whether the condition is mild, moderate, or severe; and in the latter case, whether the blood vessels, heart, or kidneys show any ill effects. The doctor will be able to discuss how the person's family history, cholesterol level, eating habits, alcohol consumption, exercise patterns, and general stress levels affect the risk of the hypertension contributing to heart disease or stroke. Based on this information, doctor and patient can work out what will be the most satisfactory course of treatment. This depends on the various factors mentioned above, and on the person's motivation to make changes in his or her life.

Treatment. Basically, the treatment for hypertension is fairly straightforward, but the *levels* at which treatment is initiated and the *type* of treatment may vary. If the average blood pressure is below 95 or 100 diastolic, the doctor may follow the person for several months, and possibly have the person take readings at home. Or the doctor may recommend lifestyle changes for a person in this range. The decision to treat with drugs will be based on whether an individual has a family history of heart attack and stroke, and whether there are any other risk factors. If the blood pressure is over 95 to 100 diastolic and the person has any significant risk factors, the doctor is more likely to prescribe antihypertensive drugs. If the blood pressure is above 100–105 diastolic, it must be lowered. In this range most doctors will start people on medication immediately.

When hypertension is not severe, some doctors may try a concerted regimen of lifestyle changes for six months. Provided the changes are successful in controlling blood pressure, the doctor may then simply monitor the person at regular intervals. But if blood pressure does not drop sufficiently, drug therapy will be started. A great many people with hypertension fall into the mild or low–moderate range and do not have significant risk factors. For these people, their *attitude* about their condition and their *motivation* to make lifestyle changes become crucial in the choice of therapy. For those people with blood pressures over 100–105 diastolic, attitude is still very important because it affects how regularly they'll take their medication, and how they'll deal with side effects if they arise. Even if drugs are prescribed, it is still important for people to pay attention to lifestyle factors. Not only can this reduce the dosages needed and even affect the choice of drugs, it will significantly lower the risks of heart attack and atherosclerotic stroke, which are the major medical problems encountered by people with high blood pressure. The decision to take control of your hypertension is the first and most important step toward better health and a longer life.

CHAPTER THREE

Hypertension and the Mind

One of the factors that plays a role in the development of high blood pressure is the way people react to stress and deal with it. It has long been known that blood pressure rises sharply when people get upset. In fact, the circulatory system has evolved to send increased amounts of blood to the voluntary muscles in response to threatening situations that require direct and immediate action. Raising blood pressure is one mechanism that helps to send blood out to the brain and muscles in an emergency. The circulatory system was designed to work efficiently when people had brief periods of challenge, stress, or danger, followed by a period of recovery and a long period of relaxation. The system does not work as well when people are under long periods of intense stress, or even under constant low levels of stress.

When people remain in an aroused state, when they face problems that they feel they cannot solve easily, their body remains in a perpetual state of alertness that eventually becomes habitual. It's as if they remain "in danger"—mentally on alert most of the time, with fewer than normal periods of recovery and relaxation. When this continues for a long period of time, blood pressure can rise and remain elevated, in a sort of Pavlovian conditioned response. Some experts theorize that artery walls eventually thicken in response to continued high blood pressure; others theorize that the pressure receptors in the carotid arteries are eventually reset so that blood pressure reaches a higher average value and doesn't return to as low a resting level. In either case, there is evidence that people can be taught to readjust their reactions to stress and learn how to truly relax. Numerous studies have shown this strategy of learning to cope with stress and to acquire relaxation skills is effective in lowering blood pressure. One of the big advantages of this approach to lowering blood pressure is that it has no side effects, as drugs sometimes do, and it can help to enhance a person's quality of life.

How stress raises blood pressure

The physiology of how stress affects blood pressure has been well documented and continues to be elaborated upon. Although the model is complex, it is useful for people to understand if they are trying to make changes in their lifestyle. At the heart of this information is the basic concept that mind and body are interconnected and continually influence each other. What we call "consciousness" or "thought" is involved with the firing of neurons in our brain, which is linked to physiological processes in the rest of the body via the spinal cord and peripheral nerves.

The nervous system consists of two parts, central and peripheral. The *central nervous system,* which is comprised of the brain and spinal cord, is made up of trillions of nerve cells connected and interconnected into circuits or loops. The brain itself is made up of the forebrain, midbrain, and hindbrain. The *forebrain* is separated into two areas, one containing the cerebral cortex and limbic system, and the other, the thalamus, hypothalamus, and pituitary gland. The *peripheral nervous system* is made up of the *somatic nervous system,* which carries impulses from the muscles and sensory receptors to and from the brain, and the *autonomic nervous system,* which carries impulses back and forth between the brain and the heart, blood vessels, and internal organs. The autonomic nervous system is responsible for continuous maintenance of the body's internal equilibrium, including heartbeat, blood pressure, hormone production, and electrolyte balance. Twenty-five years ago, these functions were thought to be purely "automatic" or involuntary; now it's known that people have a distinct degree of control over these functions.

Since the autonomic nervous system controls blood pressure, it is the key to understanding how thoughts affect blood pressure regulation. The autonomic nervous system is divided into two branches, the sympathetic and parasympathetic. The *sympathetic nervous system* moderates blood pressure both instantaneously, via the nerves that innervate the heart and the muscles in the blood vessel walls, and over a longer period of time, via stress hormones produced by the adrenal glands. Although the sympathetic nervous system is basically concerned with readying the body for quick action, it also normally sends continuous messages to small arteries throughout the body in order to maintain a low level of blood pressure that is sufficient to supply all areas of the body with blood. This minimal pressure is referred to as *vasomotor tone*.

People feel the effects of the sympathetic nervous system when they are in situations of danger, anxiety, or exertion: the heart beats faster, blood pressure rises, breathing rate increases, and blood flow is directed toward the brain and voluntary muscles. A welter of impulses from the sympathetic nervous system prepares the body for instant activity. This response, which is characterized by a pounding heart and a knot in the stomach, is referred to as the *fight-or-flight reaction*. Prolonged anxiety, which keeps the body in a constant state of sympathetic arousal, can keep the heart rate and blood pressure slightly elevated for an indefinite period. Many experts believe that over time such prolonged anxiety can cause long-term high blood pressure. They postulate that it does so in three major ways: 1) by causing the muscles in the walls of the small arteries to thicken and lose their elasticity, 2) by causing blood pressure receptors in the neck to be reset at higher levels, and 3) by affecting the salt and water balance in the kidneys.

The *parasympathetic nervous system,* in contrast, predominates when the body is at rest. It slows heart rate, causing blood pressure to drop, and redirects blood flow to the digestive organs. It is a useful simplification to say that while the sympathetic nervous system deals with danger and quick action, the parasympathetic nervous system is associated with maintenance, restoration, and healing.

The *cerebral cortex* of the brain is involved with thinking, evaluation, and awareness. It is made up of two hemispheres connected by a large bundle of nerve fibers. Researchers have found that to some degree the left side of the cerebral cortex specializes in language processing, analysis, and linear thinking, while the right side is involved with storage of images and nonverbal thought. The right hemisphere is richly connected by nerve fibers to the *limbic system,* which deals with emotions, with feelings of pleasure, pain, and anger. When a person has a thought or perception, neurons in the cerebral cortex fire and an image forms in the anterior right brain. The emotion generated by the image stimulates the limbic system, which in turn stimulates the hypothalamus and then the pituitary gland. Depending upon whether the emotion is interpreted as peaceful or upsetting, the parasympathetic or sympathetic nervous system will be activated. If the sympathetic is stimulated, heart rate increases and the arterioles constrict, a combination which causes blood pressure to go up. Over a longer period of time, the sympathetic nervous system causes the kidneys to retain sodium, which increases fluid volume, and to increase renin output, which constricts the arterioles on a more long-term basis. Both of these mechanisms contribute to a continued elevation of blood pressure.

Types of stress reactions
In recent years, doctors have found that our emotional responses to situations are usually not as simple as the fight-or-flight response. For one thing, people have different reactions to the same situation; for another, people vary in their physiological reactions to stress. Doctors have identified several types of stress reactions. First, there is a *defense reaction,* which is most like the classic fight-or-flight response. It involves elevated heart rate and increased cardiac output. Although blood pressure usually goes up, it may not go up a great deal. The rise depends upon how much the arteries leading to the voluntary muscles dilate in comparison to how much the arterioles are constricted. Animal studies have shown that frequent engagement of the defense reaction over a long period of time will eventually lead to hypertension, especially in genetically sensitive animals.

A situation that is perceived as dangerous but in which neither fight nor flight seems possible is termed a *defeat reaction*. In animals, it is typified by "playing dead"; in people, it may be the cause of fainting. A defeat reaction is characterized by frustration, depression, despair, and a sense of being overwhelmed and out of control. In this type of situation there may be an immediate slowing of the heart rate and decrease in blood pressure, but if the situation continues there may be a substantial rise in blood pressure while the heartbeat remains slow.

In modern life, people are generally less affected by physical dangers than by stressful mental situations. But whether a perceived danger is mental or physical, both a defense reaction and a defeat reaction ultimately tend to raise blood pressure. Not surprisingly, studies show that people have higher blood pressures in situations of emotional stress. For example, blood pressure tends to be higher if people have high-stress jobs, if they lose their jobs, if they live in crowded conditions, if they live in high-stress environments such as ghettos, or if there is a war (even if the people are civilians).

Relaxation

Research has demonstrated that blood pressure is a *conditioned response*, that is, a learned behavior. Both animals and humans have successfully been taught to raise or lower their blood pressure in response to a particular stimulus. In one study, animals were hooked up to measuring devices and were rewarded if their blood pressure went down. Within a short period of time, the animals learned to lower their blood pressure in order to get the desired reward. Biofeedback studies have shown that healthy individuals can learn to raise their diastolic blood pressure by as much as 20 points and lower it by as much as 10 points in response to different biofeedback cues, which is not an insignificant achievement considering that in many cases people's high blood pressure is only 10 points or so above the acceptable level.

Given the fact that blood pressure has been shown to be mediated by the autonomic nervous system, and given the fact that it has been demonstrated that people can exert some control over their blood pressure, it makes sense that people with hypertension can learn to lower their blood pressure. And, in fact, many studies done in the United States, Germany, and Russia have shown this to be true. Relaxation, meditation, biofeedback, yoga, hypnosis, and Autogenic Training have all been shown to lower blood pressure over a period of time. All of these methods have in common learning a technique that leads to a reduction of sympathetic nervous system arousal and produces a state of relaxation. Many researchers feel that such "arousal reduction treatments" are especially beneficial as an alternative to drug therapy for people who have mild-to-moderate hypertension, since relaxation techniques have no negative side effects and they cost less than long-term drug therapy. In Germany, such treatments have been so successful in eliminating the need for drugs in people with mild high blood pressure that they are also being used to treat moderate hypertension.

In a review of 18 studies, relaxation techniques were found to lower systolic pressure by 11 points, and diastolic pressure by 7 points in people who had recently been taught the techniques. Doctors theorize that people who are very motivated and practice these techniques over a long period of time may be able to achieve and maintain even greater reductions. Studies in Russia and Germany on relaxation techniques have indicated that motivated people with moderate hypertension have been able to lower their blood pressure enough to go off medication. Studies like this have not yet been done in the U.S.

Stress, attitude, and personality

Another link between stress and high blood pressure is that people with hypertension show greater blood pressure increases in response to stress than do people with normal blood pressure. Likewise, children who have normal blood pressure but whose parents have hypertension show a greater response to stress than children who do not have a family history of hypertension. This has led researchers to theorize that the behavioral response to stress may be different in people who become hypertensive, that these people perceive challenges differently and react in a more emotional manner. At present, researchers do not know whether this is the result of an *inherited* tendency or a *learned* behavioral style. In either case, it underscores how important it is for people with hypertension to learn a different style of reacting, a new way of coping with stress.

Extensive work on hypertension and coping has been done in Germany and Russia, where relaxation instruction is paired with psychotherapeutic techniques for coping. This work has led to a more holistic view of hypertension. The aim is not only to relax muscles, but to change the way people perceive the world. This holistic view of hypertension has been corroborated by American studies which found that relaxation techniques were effective in lowering blood pressure even in people who did not demonstrate "relaxation" in their muscles, and who did not do their exercises regularly. The doctors who conducted these studies theorized that the drop in blood pressure was not so much a matter of relaxation as a change in attitude.

These findings fit in with the recent research on stress. Stress is no longer thought to be simply an external problem or situation; rather, stress lies in the way people perceive an event or situation and whether or not they believe they can cope with it. The most widely accepted theory on stress stems from the work of psychologist Richard Lazarus. Lazarus hypothesizes that when people experience any life event, they appraise the situation in order to see if they need to act on it, and if so, they then assess whether or not they have the resources to deal with the problem. In effect, people are always weighing the need to act against the ability to cope. Based on their own appraisal, people view events as either a challenge that they can successfully meet, or a threat that may have a negative outcome. If they perceive a situation as somehow threatening, they experience stress and their body reacts by raising their blood pressure until such time as the stress is resolved.

Stanford psychologist Albert Bandura has termed people's perception of their ability to cope *self-efficacy*. He found that people with low

ATTITUDES THAT HELP TO PROMOTE HEALTH AND LOWER BLOOD PRESSURE

Self-efficacy: a perception that one is able to cope.
Hardiness: a clear sense of values, and a sense of control.
Coherence: confidence that the world is predictable and life will work out reasonably.

self-efficacy felt stress in study situations and showed high levels of stress hormones in their blood. After training these people to develop a measure of control over a specific stressful situation, he found that they could do the same task with no perception of stress and no increase in stress hormones. The implications of this study are far-reaching. It shows that when people change their perception of their ability to cope with stress, their physiological response changes. Logically, one can predict that blood pressure would be lower as well.

Other researchers have dealt with the question of whether or not there are personality characteristics that help people cope more effectively with stressful situations. Social psychologist Suzanne Kobasa studied a large number of executives during a time of restructuring within their company. She found that one group became ill, while another did not. The two groups were matched sociologically, and differed only in personality. She termed the personality type of the healthy group "hardiness." She divided hardiness into three interrelated components: control, commitment, and challenge. By *control*, Kobasa meant a belief that one can influence the events taking place around oneself. The opposite of control is helplessness. *Commitment* relates to active involvement in one's life, and a sense of purpose about life. The opposite of commitment is alienation and a sense of meaninglessness. The third component, *challenge*, involves seeing a situation as a problem to be solved rather than an insurmountable threat of which one is a victim. Challenge implies a belief in one's ability to change a situation.

Israeli medical sociologist Aaron Antonovsky looks at coping qualities not as a personality type, but as a philosophy or world outlook. He terms a health-producing outlook a *sense of coherence*. Such a philosophy involves seeing life events as opportunities, not threats.

COHERENCE FACTORS THAT PROMOTE HEALTH

Comprehensibility: the world appears orderly, the future seems predictable.

Manageability: a feeling that one can cope.

Meaningfulness: a sense of emotional involvement in one's experiences.

Antonovsky divides coherence into three parts: comprehensibility, manageability, and meaningfulness. By *comprehensibility* he means that the world is understandable and somewhat predictable; it does not necessarily imply that a situation is either good or bad; rather, that it is "known." The opposite of this characteristic is chaos, that is, a situation that simply does not make sense. *Manageability* involves a sense that one can meet the demands required by a given situation, either alone or by getting help. The opposite of manageability is helplessness. The third aspect of a sense of coherence is *meaningfulness,* that is, that a given situation is important, and that one is involved in its outcome. The opposite of meaningfulness is apathy or lack of interest. Antonovsky feels that when people have a strong sense of coherence to their lives, they have a reason to be healthy, and they believe that their actions can produce desired results. He thinks that such people are more likely to adopt health-promoting lifestyles and to solve problems rather than be overcome by them.

Coping with stress

There are basically two ways to cope with stress: first, people can work to prevent or reduce the stress; secondly, they can improve their ability to deal with stress. An example of the first approach would be if commuters who always became anxious that traffic congestion might make them late to work decided to take the train instead of driving. An example of the second approach would be if they practiced relaxation during the drive to work. The second approach is more applicable to life problems in which the stress cannot readily be eliminated. Coping skills can be strengthened by increasing one's support and by learning such techniques as meditation, relaxation, and imagery. People can also work to change their attitudes and outlook on the world. Some people are able to do this by themselves, others find they are more productive if they work with a counselor or therapist.

Support

Studies have shown that support is very effective in countering the negative effects of stress. Support can broadly be defined as anything that makes people feel good, function more effectively, and/or feel

CHARACTERISTICS OF PEOPLE WHO GET ILL, AND PEOPLE WHO DON'T

Likely to become ill	Less likely to become ill
Crisis-ridden	Optimistic
Under stress	Has a purpose in life, a reason for being
Dissatisfied	
Unhappy	Trusting
Resentful	High self-esteem
Threatened	Gets along well with peers
Out of control	Successful
Loaded with responsibility	Excited
Worried	Interested
Depressed	Satisfied
Frustrated	Stimulated
Helpless	Happy
Lonely	Involved
Grief-stricken	Part of stable social structure
Confused	Has sense of cohesion
Lacks positive feedback	Has social support, positive feedback

more optimistic. It leads people to have a sense of being loved, nourished, and satisfied; it raises their self-esteem and makes them feel part of something larger than themselves. Self-esteem produces increased hardiness and a greater sense of coherence. Support can come from close relationships with family and friends, from jobs or hobbies that give people positive feedback, and from belief systems or religions that give meaning to life. In terms of hypertension, support may (or may not) come from a person's family, friends, and doctor. Support has even been shown to affect longevity. In the Alameda County study, Lisa

SIGNS OF SIGNIFICANT STRESS

Tension, anxiety

Agitation, restlessness, inability to relax

Constant worrying

Sense of time pressure

Inability to concentrate

Apathy, sadness

Feelings of insecurity or worthlessness

Feelings of powerlessness or inability to cope

Frequent irritability, argumentativeness, and/or anger

Defensiveness

Arrogance, grandiosity

Procrastination, chronic lateness

Chronic fatigue

Lack of sexual interest

Sexual promiscuity

Poor appearance

Legal problems

Frequent illnesses or accidents

Crying spells

Nervous indigestion

Compulsive eating

Compulsive smoking

Headaches

Neck and shoulder pain

Use of tranquilizers or recreational drugs to relax

Berkman and Lester Breslow found that people who were married, had close contacts with friends or relatives, or had associations with church or nonchurch groups showed lower mortality rates than people who did not have these supports. It is interesting to note that the *degree of intimacy* involved was more important than the *type of relationship*.

In terms of hypertension, there are a number of specific ways in which support can play an important role. First, a general sense of feeling loved and secure makes people feel safer and worry less, which helps to lower their overall state of sympathetic arousal. A person with hypertension can work to make his or her feelings and needs for support known to others; at the same time, relatives, friends, and medical personnel can demonstrate their concern and be sensitive to the person's needs. From a practical standpoint, it's important that a person with hypertension express his or her concerns and worries to the doctor, family members, and friends. The more family members understand about high blood pressure and its treatment, the more supportive they will be able to be. Family members can help the person with hypertension undertake and maintain healthy lifestyle changes by reducing household stress; supporting a low-salt, low-fat diet; helping with weight reduction if it is recommended; and encouraging the person to exercise.

Setting coping goals

In terms of stress reduction, there is much that people with hypertension can do. The first thing is for people to become more aware of what

---

WHY SOCIAL SUPPORT INCREASES HEALTH

- It gratifies emotional needs for security, affection, trust, intimacy, nurturing, a sense of belonging.
- It helps in appraising and defining reality.
- It makes people aware of shared norms of feeling and behavior.
- It increases group solidarity.
- It increases self-esteem through social approval.

EVALUATING SUPPORT

1. Do you confide in someone each day, once a week, less than once a week, never?
2. Do you feel secure in your environment each day, once a week, less than once a week, never?
3. Do you feel that you have some control over your environment each day, once a week, less than once a week, never?
4. Do you feel that people approve of you each day, once a week, less than once a week, never?
5. Does your support come from family, friends, groups, and/or community?
6. Do you feel that you have enough money? Usually? Sometimes? Never?
7. Do you have a strong set of personal beliefs? A strong religious affiliation?

is stressful in their lives, and to make a plan to reduce the stress. This requires an ongoing examination of work, school, family relationships, finances, and leisure activities. People should also look at recent life events that have required change or adjustment. Seattle psychiatrists Thomas Holmes and Richard Rahe found that life events—even positive ones—that required change and adaptation were stress producing. This is especially true of changes that involve a person's closest relationships or financial pressures. Most people find it is useful to list the stresses, and then categorize them according to whether they can be

STEPS TO REDUCING LIFE STRESS

1. Identify major stressors: e.g., financial problems, marital problems, death in family, too many deadlines, overbooked schedule, lack of support.
2. Set short- and long-term goals.
3. Begin by changing the stresses that are easiest to deal with.
4. Do something to lower stress and/or feel good each day.
5. Get help with problems that are difficult to deal with by yourself.

dealt with immediately, at a later time, or are unchangeable. Being late for work is an example of a stress that can be dealt with rather directly. Leaving a stressful job for a more fulfilling one is not unrealistic, but it may take some time to accomplish. A divorce or death is an event that can be dealt with, but cannot be changed. After identifying external stresses and categorizing them, people need to set realistic goals, both short- and long-term, to deal with those stresses which can be changed. Likewise, people can identify those stressful areas that cannot be changed and see how a different attitude might make it easier to cope with them.

In addition to dealing with stresses in the outside world, it's important to deal with internal issues, that is, attitudes and life views. This is often more difficult because people are less aware of their own psychological states, and attitudes are often resistant to change. The first step is to become aware of what you are thinking about when you feel uncomfortable. In time, people often notice that they have certain feelings under the surface that come up over and over, or arise in different situations. Such feelings may involve conflicts with other people, fears and worries about the past or future, or negative feelings about themselves. These kinds of issues are difficult for anyone to face. You may find you say "No problem," or "I don't mind" when you are actually irritated with someone, or you may become angry at others or

---

ACTIVITIES THAT HELP TO LOWER STRESS

- Discussing your concerns with friends.
- Doing something nice for yourself each day.
- Exercising at least 15–30 minutes 3–5 times a week.
- Getting enough rest—going to bed early, or catnapping during the afternoon or commute time.
- Meditating 15–20 minutes a day.
- Practicing relaxation or imagery exercises 15–20 minutes a day.
- Engaging in hobbies or relaxing activities such as walking, gardening, or listening to music.
- Changing your pace and/or your routines.
- Getting outside help when the stress level is too great.

---

sad within yourself when you feel in some way inadequate. Once you become aware of areas of conflict, fear, or negativity, the next step is simply to *observe yourself without judgment* to learn more about yourself. In order to bring about lasting change, you have to accept yourself and be compassionate toward yourself. The last step is to share your feelings with friends. Often they will have had similar feelings, and will give you support and validation.

One of the most important issues in getting support is to improve personal communication skills. Often a person avoids expressing personal needs directly (*passive communication*), and then feels resentful when those needs are not met. Conversely, another person might attack others, or threaten them (*aggressive communication*) when he or she wants something done. As a result, people avoid the person. Better communication can be established by expressing feelings honestly and openly, and standing up for oneself. This is called *assertive communication*. At the core of it is a respect for other people's feelings as well as your own. If you cannot make headway with personal problems, seek help from a trained counselor. Unresolved, deep-seated issues are thought to contribute to hypertension in many people by keeping them in a constant state of stress. Several studies have shown that in some people psychotherapy can reduce blood pressure.

How relaxation affects blood pressure

Relaxation techniques lower blood pressure by directly reducing sympathetic arousal. The physiology of the relaxation response is the op-

---

BECOMING AWARE OF MUSCLE TENSION

To feel muscle tension, lie in a comfortable position with your hands resting at your sides. Raise one hand slightly by bending it at the wrist; you will feel the muscles in the top of your forearm contract and tense. If you let your hand go limp, these muscles will relax and your hand will drop. With practice, you will become aware of the subtle difference in feeling between a contracted muscle and a relaxed one. If you're not sure of the feeling of tension, rest the fingers of your other hand lightly on top of your forearm and feel the muscle contract as you raise your hand.

TENSION SPOTS

Everyone has certain areas or muscles that become tense when he or she is nervous or under pressure. These are the most common areas to check for tension:
- Eyes
- Jaw
- Neck and shoulders
- Lower back and pelvis

posite of the physiological mechanism that causes high blood pressure. When a person is relaxed, messages from the hypothalamus quiet the sympathetic branch of the nervous system and stimulate the parasympathetic branch. As a result, heart rate drops, cardiac output decreases, and the smooth muscles in the arterioles relax. Due to the decrease in both cardiac output and peripheral resistance, blood pressure drops.

Relaxation is a process that involves turning inward and concentrating on the inner world rather than the external world. People relax in many ways—by listening to music, lying in the sun, gardening, or exercising. These are goal-less activities in that they are not oriented toward solving a problem or achieving an immediate result. They automatically remove people from a situation in which they must appraise their own ability to act.

Relaxation techniques move the body into a deeply relaxed state in a more direct way than hobbies or leisure activities, but it is important to realize that you do not *do* relaxation, you *allow* it to happen. The feeling of relaxation is a natural one that takes place when tension is removed. There are many methods for learning relaxation, all of which are effective. They have in common a clear set of instructions, a comfortable position, a passive attitude of allowing relaxation to take place, a quiet place in which to be undisturbed, and a deep, regular breathing rate. *Autosuggestion,* one of the most popular techniques, involves hearing or reading directions and mentally repeating them. The specific words are not important; what is, is letting your body relax.

BASIC RELAXATION

Find a comfortable space where you will not be disturbed. Sit or lie down with your legs uncrossed, your arms at your sides or resting on your abdomen. Loosen any tight or constricting clothing. Close your eyes. Begin by inhaling slowly and deeply through your nostrils. Let the breath out slowly and completely. Continue breathing in this manner, allowing your abdomen to rise as you inhale, and fall as you exhale. As you breathe, allow yourself to relax. Let your consciousness float behind your nostrils and feel the air going in and out of your nose. Now shift your consciousness to your feet, and allow them to relax. Concentrate on feelings of tingling, buzzing, pulsing, warmth or coolness, heaviness or lightness. Now let your ankles relax. Allow the feelings of relaxation to spread up the backs of your legs. Now allow your calves to relax. Continue to breathe in and out slowly, and let the feelings of relaxation deepen. Allow your knees to relax, and the muscles of your thighs. While you're relaxing, let your mind float free, momentarily alighting on the feeling of air moving through your nostrils, then concentrating on the particular part of your body you are relaxing. Take a moment and release any worries or anxieties you may have. Release them—you don't need them—and let them drift away. If you wish, you may watch them float off as you exhale. You can name the particular worry, and see it slip away as a bubble, a dark area, or a bird. All you're doing here is allowing your body to relax, which it knows how to do by itself.

Now allow your pelvic area to relax. Feel the relaxation in your genitals, anus, and buttocks. Release the tension that everyone carries in their pelvis. Now let your abdomen relax. Allow it to relax as it rises and falls; allow your breathing to take place by itself. Allow the muscles of your chest to relax. Let your breath go in and out smoothly; allow your breathing to take place by itself. Let your heartbeat be smooth and regular. Let your mind float over your entire body. Concentrate on feelings of buzzing, vibrating, tingling, lightness or heaviness. You may notice that your body feels as if it were getting larger or that space seems to be expanding. You may also notice that the inside of your body seems hollow and large, and that your entire consciousness seems quiet and deep.

Allow the feelings of relaxation that you are experiencing to spread into your shoulders. Let your shoulders relax; let them drop. Now let your upper arms relax, and let the feeling spread to your lower arms and hands. Feel the sensations of tingling and numbness spread through your hands, and let your mind wander back over your body, down to your feet, deepening the relaxation throughout your whole body. Now let your neck relax. Let the big muscles that support your head loosen and lengthen. Now let the feelings of relaxation spread up to your head. Relax your scalp, let your jaw drop, let the muscles around your eyes relax, and let your forehead relax.

Now concentrate on a place on the top of your head. You may feel tingling or buzz-

BASIC RELAXATION (cont.)

ing there. As you take a breath, allow energy to flow into your body through that area, and allow your body to expand. Imagine that millions of moving particles of light come into your body through the top of your head, go down along your spine, and out and around to envelop your whole body. Enjoy these feelings of relaxation. It almost seems as if your body disappears, and your consciousness is floating outside your body, in front of your eyes. Now direct your attention to any areas of your body that feel tense or that bother you. Let them relax; let them drop. Allow the energy coming in through your head to flow to those areas, move around them, and caress them. Allow the energy to go through them and fill them with light. Remain in this wonderfully relaxed state as long as you wish.

When you wish to return to your everyday state, gently move your feet and count slowly from one to three. You will return to your everyday state relaxed, comfortable, and full of energy. Your body will feel like it is in a comfortable healing space. Each time you do this exercise, you will relax more deeply and more easily. The feelings of relaxation will deepen, and the whole exercise will become more and more pleasurable.

When the body relaxes, muscle fibers actually become longer, heart and metabolic rate drop, brain wave patterns change, and the levels of stress hormones decrease. These physical signs of relaxation are accompanied by changes in a person's mental state. Relaxation produces an altered state of consciousness called the *reverie state*. Time and space appear differently, logical thinking is replaced by more immediate, feeling-oriented thinking, and people experience an increased sense

WHEN TO USE RELAXATION

Relax your body and mind completely:
- when you are worried.
- when you are upset, angry, or unhappy.
- when you feel stressed.
- when you are very tired.
- when you feel you are getting sick.
- when some part of your body hurts.
- just to make yourself feel good.

of oneness with the world around them. People often notice sensations such as tingling, numbness, lightness or heaviness, which make them aware of the fact that their body is functioning by itself. Relaxation spontaneously brings about changes in people's attitudes; it counters fears, anger, worries, and sadness. At the same time, it enhances feelings of pleasure, self-acceptance, connectedness, and control. Studies have shown that blood pressure not only drops during relaxation exercises, it stays down for a period of time afterward, affecting the way that people react to stress. This happens whether or not their muscles relax or their stress hormones decrease. Apparently, what's most important is the change in a person's mental state.

How meditation affects blood pressure

For thousands of years, meditation has been used to focus the mind, relax the body, and quiet the spirit. Several forms of meditation have been studied in relation to hypertension, and have been found to be effective in lowering blood pressure. Using meditation techniques, yogis have shown that they can voluntarily control important physiological functions: they are able to slow their heart rate and raise their skin temperature at will.

Herbert Benson, from the Harvard Department of Behavioral Medicine, has perfected an exercise, based on transcendental meditation, which induces a physiological state he calls the *relaxation response.* Like relaxation exercises, his meditation exercise involves a process of going inward and letting go, reducing goal-striving activity. The result is a quieting of the sympathetic nervous system. Benson's meditation exercise causes a drop in heart rate, breathing rate, blood pressure, and a shift in brain waves from alert *beta* to relaxed *alpha* rhythms.

Most types of meditation involve simply keeping the mind focused on the present moment. To facilitate this endeavor, meditation techniques have people count their breaths, pay attention to their breathing, or repeat a word, number, or phrase over and over with each breath. In Eastern religions, these words are referred to as *mantras,* and they have a spiritual meaning. The two most famous ones are "om," believed to be the primordial sound, and "ham sah," which means "I am that." One of the basic concepts of meditation is that people should

A MEDITATION EXERCISE

Find a tranquil place where you won't be disturbed. Sit in a comfortable position with your back straight but relaxed. Close your eyes. Inhale slowly and deeply, then exhale slowly and completely. As you breathe in and out, allow your body to relax. Breathe naturally, and become aware of your breath as it enters your nostrils. As you breathe, keep your attention on this area of your nose, and feel the sensations as each breath flows in and out. Maintain your attention on your breathing. If an outside thought, sensation, or sound enters your mind, note it for what it is ("thinking," "sound," or "sensation") without passing judgment, and return your attention to the breath in your nostrils. Continue to breathe naturally and keep your body relaxed. Imagine that you are like a watchman at a gate, who simply notes what passes in and out, but does not follow it. Whenever your mind wanders off and you lose track, simply return your awareness to your breathing.

Do this exercise for 15–20 minutes, once or twice a day. Initially you may want to set a timer in another room or just check your watch when you think 15–20 minutes have passed. Don't be concerned about how *well* you meditate. The point of the exercise is simply to keep your mind focused on your breathing for the allotted time period. Everyone's mind wanders. The goal is not to hold onto your thoughts, but to be aware of your breathing. Some people find that it helps to say a word or mantra such as "om," "Lord," or "peace" as they inhale and exhale. Alternatively, some people mentally say "one" or "in" as they inhale, and "two" or "out" as they exhale. The point is to focus; it's not so important what you focus on.

not be concerned about how they're doing—about their success or failure in maintaining their counting or repeating a particular phrase. Everyone's mind wanders; that is to be expected. The task is simply to return to the count or phrase whenever the mind does stray. For most people, beginning to meditate is a revelation. They have never realized that so many diverse thoughts go through their mind continuously, or that they have so little control over their own thoughts.

In terms of hypertension, meditation has several specific uses that are important. First, as we've said, it quiets the sympathetic nervous system, thereby lowering blood pressure during the period of meditation, and for a variable period of time afterward. Second, by helping people to become aware of what's going through their mind and gain a measure of control over their thoughts, meditation helps people cope with stress, worry, and fear. This change helps to quiet the sympathetic nervous system on a continuing basis, which tends to lower blood pressure over a long period of time. Finally, as the yogis were aware, meditation can lead to a degree of inner peace or enlightenment that adds to the comprehensibility and meaningfulness of life. This shift in attitude may ultimately be the most important long-term effect of meditation, being even more valuable than an immediate reduction in blood pressure.

How imagery affects blood pressure

Imagery is a process that involves picturing scenes or events in the mind's eye. People visualize all the time, often without realizing it. They picture events from the past, set goals for the future, and envision solutions to problems in their life or work. In spite of the fact that most people image constantly, they rarely make conscious use of this skill. Seeing with the mind's eye is an inner process that is both similar to, and different from, experiences in the outer world. Like outer-world experiences, imagery can involve all the senses. *Unlike* experiences in the outer world, imagery involves concentrating on a thought or idea.

Imagery's value in treating hypertension stems from two basic effects. First, the body responds to imagery physiologically in a manner similar to the way it responds to outer events. For example, if you imagine being at rest in a place that you love, your heart beats more slowly and your blood pressure drops, just as if you were actually there. The images held in the frontal lobes of the cerebral hemispheres cause nerve impulses to go to the hypothalamus in the back of the brain, which in turn quiets the sympathetic nervous system. Second, imagery is valuable in treating hypertension because images affect people's outlook. Often images that arise spontaneously appear as symbols from our deepest self. Such symbols can help people grow and achieve greater self-knowledge and a sense of basic fulfillment. Imagery is used in counseling to change people's attitudes and promote self-esteem, self-efficacy, and personal growth.

BEGINNING IMAGERY

Find a comfortable space where you will not be disturbed. Sit or lie down with your legs uncrossed, your arms at your sides or resting on your abdomen. Loosen any tight or constricting clothing. Close your eyes. Begin by inhaling slowly and deeply through your nostrils. Let the breath out slowly and completely. Continue breathing in this manner, allowing your abdomen to rise as you inhale, and fall as you exhale. As you breathe, allow yourself to relax. Let yourself relax completely. Release any worries or tensions that you have; let them float off. Let the feeling of relaxation spread throughout your body. (If you feel it is necessary, repeat the Basic Relaxation exercise on page 53.

Now imagine that you are in a comfortable room. It may be a room in the place where you live, work, or grew up. Imagine that you are in the middle of the room on a bright sunny day. Give yourself a moment to get used to your surroundings. Glance around the room. Notice the doors, the windows, the floor, the ceiling, and any furniture in the room. Let your eyes take in the objects in the room; scan them. Now mentally zoom in on any piece of furniture, and concentrate on the details. Look at what it is made of, its style and carving. Look at the surface; now touch it and feel its texture. Is it rough or smooth, warm or cold? Now zoom in on other objects in your room. See what the windowsills and curtains are made of. Look closely at the other furniture. Let your eyes travel and take in details. Notice scratches or chips in paint, light reflections, and shiny areas. Touch the windowsill or furniture. Feel the texture of the material from which they are made. Smell the air in the room. Does it have a particular odor of wood, perfume, or flowers? Listen for any sounds in the room. Is there a clock ticking, are there noises coming from the rest of the house or from outside? Get as vivid a picture of the room as you can.

Now, in your mind's eye, imagine making changes in the room. Because this is in your imagination, you can make any changes you wish. First, mentally rearrange the furniture. Try the furniture in a number of different locations. If you wish, remove some of the furniture entirely or add new pieces. Now imagine that the walls of the room change color. Choose any colors or wallpaper that you wish. Also, imagine that the floor is different. Pick any kind of rug, hardwood floor, or tile. Each time you make a change, you can make it turn back, or you can keep it. Now imagine that the windows or doors change shape or position. You might make the windows larger or move them to a different place on the wall; you might make them out of a different material or architectural style. Finally, you might change the shape or size of the room. You could expand the room, make it round, or change the ceiling. Make changes in your room for as long as you wish.

Now let your room return to its original state. Pause a moment and look around. Get comfortable. Then imagine that someone you love or respect, a

BEGINNING IMAGERY (cont.)

family member or close friend, is coming to visit you in your room. You can invite anyone you wish, or let the person who comes be a surprise to you. Look up when that person knocks at the door, and watch as he or she enters the room. Notice what the person is wearing and how he or she walks. Greet the person, and listen for a reply. Begin a conversation. Tell the person that you're happy to see him or her, and talk as if the person really was in the room with you. When you finish speaking, pause and hear what the person says in return. It will seem to you like the other side of an inner conversation with yourself. You can talk about a shared interest or ask any questions you wish. You may want to tell the person something that you haven't been able to share before. Continue the conversation as long as you wish. Say good-by and watch as the person leaves your room.

Now imagine that your room undergoes a radical change, and becomes a place to begin a journey. Let all the furniture disappear. Let the ceiling and the roof lift off, exposing the sky. Let the walls fold out. You are now on a platform with the sky above you. Imagine that you start to float upward from the platform, rising at a faster and faster speed until you are soaring. The space around you is now turning dark and stars begin to appear. Continue rising into the dark, starry sky. In front of you, in the distance, you will see an area of white light. The area is bright, but so far away that it appears to be only several feet in diameter. Allow yourself to drift toward the light. Notice the stars moving past you as you drift. As you move toward it, the area of white light becomes larger and larger. Finally, it begins to fill your whole field. Allow yourself to drift into the center of the light. Feel the light around you. Imagine the light is made up of millions of dots of moving energy. Imagine that the dots of energy can move through your body easily, as if it were not solid. Now feel the light and energy inside you, as well as around you. Feel yourself become one with the light and its energy. If any areas of your body attract your attention, allow the light and energy to increase there. Rest in the healing peace of the light as long as you wish.

When you wish to return to your everyday state, gently move your feet and count slowly from one to three. You will return to your everyday state, relaxed, comfortable, and full of energy. Your body will feel like it is in a comfortable healing space. Each time you do this exercise, you will relax more deeply and more easily. The feelings of relaxation will deepen, and the whole exercise will become more and more pleasurable.

IMAGERY FOR HEALING

First do the Basic Relaxation exercise (see page 53) to get yourself in a deeply relaxed state.

For any illness:
- When relaxed, first picture your illness, then let the image of your illness turn into an image of healing.
- Images that come from inside you are often the most vivid and powerful. Let go of images that make you frightened or uncomfortable.
- Your images may be anatomical, symbolic, poetic, cartoonlike, etc., and may involve any or all of your senses. You can make use of the anatomical and physiological information given in the text.
- Picture the area bathed in white light; picture healing energy going to the injured area; picture the area as completely healed.
- Imagine tension and pain leaving your body as you breathe out.
- Imagine healthy immune cells engulfing bacteria or virus.
- Imagine blood flow increasing to an injured area; imagine drugs getting in to heal an area or relieve the pain.
- Imagine your body replacing damaged cells with new healthy cells.
- Imagine the swelling in an area decreasing.
- Imagine rough areas as smooth, hot areas as cool, and dry areas as moist.
- Picture yourself active, healthy, relaxed, and involved in activities you enjoy.

For specific illnesses:
- For *heart disease,* picture your coronary arteries as smooth and open, easily bringing blood to all parts of the heart.
- For *high blood pressure,* picture all your blood vessels relaxing and imagine the blood flowing smoothly and easily throughout your body.

In terms of use, we separate imagery into two categories, receptive and programmed. *Receptive imagery* involves clearing the mind and letting images arise spontaneously. Through receptive imagery, people can identify positive and negative feelings about their life, job, family, and outside interests. This process can help people bring important ideas and concerns to consciousness, and help them deal more effec-

AN EXERCISE FOR GETTING A SPIRIT GUIDE

Find a quite space where you will be undisturbed, a place where you will feel at ease. Make yourself comfortable. Close your eyes. Inhale slowly and deeply; exhale slowly and completely. As you breathe in and out, allow your body to relax very deeply. Allow your abdomen to rise and fall as you breathe. Breathe in, and as you exhale, slowly say to yourself, "Three, three, three." See the numeral or the word *three* as you repeat it. Inhale again, and as you exhale, repeat and visualize the number *two*. Inhale again, and as you exhale, repeat and visualize the number *one*.

You are now in a calm and relaxed state of being; you can deepen this state by counting backward. Breathe in. As you exhale, say to yourself, "Ten, I am feeling very relaxed." Inhale again and as you exhale repeat mentally, "Nine, I am feeling more relaxed." Breathe. "Eight, I am feeling even more relaxed. Seven, deeper and more relaxed. Six, more relaxed. Five, deeper and more relaxed. Four, deeper and more relaxed. Three, deeper and more relaxed. Two, deeper and more relaxed. One, deeper and more relaxed."

You are now at a deeper and more relaxed level of awareness, a level where you feel healthy, peaceful, and open. Allow yourself to picture a place or a room where you can work in your inner world. The room can be as real as a studio, shop, or meadow, but it exists in your mind. Begin to look around. Notice whether you are outdoors or in a room. If you are in a room, notice how the walls, doors, and windows look. If you are out of doors, look closely at the trees, plants, and rocks. Because you are visualizing this space, there are no limits to what you may see in it. In this imaginary protected space, you can meet an inner guide.

If you are inside, imagine a special door which slides open from the bottom to the top. Allow the door to slide open slowly. First you will see the guide's feet, then the legs, then the entire body. The guide may be a man or a woman, an animal or a plant, a strange being, or even a light or sound. Now ask the guide to communicate with you. You can even ask the guide's name and talk to the guide. If the guide begins to speak, let the information flow into your mind. It will sound like an inner conversation, but the guide's voice will be spontaneous. Ask the guide if you can talk further, and ask any questions about your life and health. Stay with your guide in your inner space as long as you wish. When you are ready to return to your ordinary state, count slowly from one to three and gently

AN EXERCISE FOR GETTING A SPIRIT GUIDE (cont.)

move some part of your body. Slowly allow yourself to return to your everyday consciousness and open your eyes when you are ready to do so. You will feel rested and calm and will be able to return to your inner world and guide whenever you wish.

tively with problems in their life. People can even use receptive imagery to get in touch with specific symbols of their illness and the means to heal it. A specialized form of receptive imagery involves meeting and talking with an inner voice, advisor, or guide. Such inner figures have been used by Native Americans for centuries. Psychiatrist Carl Jung used inner guides as part of his *active imagination therapy.* Jung considers the inner voice to be part of the subconscious. Native Americans saw the inner voice as a spirit. In any case, people use an inner voice by having a conversation with themselves, like an inner dialogue. In dealing with hypertension, inner guides can give advice on ways to relieve personal stress and make life more fulfilling.

Programmed imagery involves choosing and holding particular images, either ones that have been suggested, or personal ones that arise during receptive imagery. Programmed imagery is the most common type used in healing physical illnesses; using images that come from your own imagination is generally the most powerful. An example of programmed imagery for hypertension would be to picture blood ves-

**HOW TO USE RECEPTIVE IMAGERY TO GET IN TOUCH
WITH INNER FEELINGS**

1. Visualize how you'd like to spend your time at work, at home.
2. Visualize how you'd like family relationships to be—how you'd like your children and partner to treat you, how you'd like to treat them.
3. Visualize the most pleasurable family vacation or weekend that you can imagine.
4. Visualize things that you could do to improve problem areas in your personal life, your family life, your work.
5. Visualize situations that make you or family members sick or healthy.

sels widening and blood flowing more smoothly and easily. Programmed imagery may involve biological or symbolic images, or a mixture of the two. The image of blood vessels widening is biological in nature. A symbolic or metaphorical image related to blood pressure might be a flower opening up or a river widening and becoming calmer on its way to the sea. Psychologists and doctors who work with imagery often have people draw a picture of their illness, then ask them to visualize and draw another picture showing how forces from inside or outside their body might heal the illness. During this process, many people find that the initial images that come to mind are anatomical in nature, but later the images often become more symbolic. In dealing specifically with hypertension, people may find it helpful to work with the physiological information given in the previous chapter and in the chapter on drugs. For example, people might picture the smooth muscle cells in their arterioles relaxing, or they might visualize their kidneys excreting more water. The most important thing is to make the images as vivid as possible. When the images become "real," even if only momentarily, they have great power.

Imagery is not a static process, it's dynamic. Generally people don't see one fixed image, they see a series of images that form a process. Working with healing imagery is usually not like looking at a still photograph, rather it is like looking at a movie. The succession of images that come from deep inside are receptive images; the ones we choose to concentrate on and elaborate on are programmed images. The process that we image is the physiology of healing. When we picture healing in our minds, it helps healing to take place in our body.

Getting help

All stress reduction techniques can be done alone, or with a counselor or therapist. Based on the theory that stress plays a fundamental role in the development and maintenance of hypertension, it makes sense that either group or individual work with a counselor might be an effective primary treatment that could reduce or eliminate the need for antihypertensive drugs in many people. Stress reduction has not been a major focus of treatment in this country, but it has been in European countries and the U.S.S.R. In those countries it has been used successfully without drugs to control mild and moderate hypertension. In the U.S., doctors have concentrated more on drug and dietary therapies.

Some people find they can readily employ stress reduction therapies they read about in books. Others find they need workshops, classes, or individual counseling to get started with these techniques and utilize them most effectively. Due to the public interest in and growth of behavioral medicine, there are now a number of professionals who can train people in relaxation techniques. Psychologists, family counselors, social workers, and nurses work with both groups and individuals. They may use relaxation, biofeedback, meditation, imagery, or hypnosis, in addition to helping people deal with internal issues or life problems. Generally, instruction in some basic stress reduction technique, such as hypnosis, requires five to ten sessions. A drop in blood pressure is often noticed within several sessions, and continues after the sessions stop, provided people continue to react to stressful situations with less arousal.

CHAPTER FOUR

Hypertension and Diet

Doctors have known for many years that a number of dietary factors are associated with hypertension. Recent research has shown that losing weight and lowering salt, fat, and alcohol intake have a positive effect on lowering blood pressure. Increasing the intake of potassium, calcium, and fiber also helps to lower blood pressure. Thus, there is much that people with hypertension can do to lower their blood pressure through dietary means.

The earliest association to be demonstrated between hypertension and diet involved the consumption of salt. Hundreds of studies have shown that cultures with a low-salt diet have virtually no high blood pressure, whereas hypertension is most common in cultures with a high-salt diet. In the early years of hypertension research, physiologists were searching for a single isolated cause of high blood pressure, and many researchers believed that salt alone raised blood pressure by causing the kidneys to retain fluid, thereby increasing blood volume. Studies on the Yanamamo Indians of the Amazon and the Eskimos of Alaska, both of whom had very low-salt diets, revealed almost no incidence of hypertension, stroke, or heart attack. By comparison, the people of northern Japan, whose diet included soy sauce, miso soup, and pickled vegetables, had the highest incidence of hypertension in the world (over 60%), and their major cause of death was stroke. Subsequently, in response to two government programs that successfully caused people to alter their diet, the incidence of hypertension and stroke declined significantly in that area of Japan.

Until the 1950s, dietary intervention was the only medical treatment for hypertension. The most famous, and the most radical, treatment was the Kempner Diet. Dr. Walter Kempner of North Carolina found that he was able to control severe high blood pressure with a diet of boiled rice and fruit. Although this treatment was successful, most Americans in the 1950s were unwilling to limit their diet so severely. Unfortunately, many people lumped all dietary treatment with the Kempner Diet, which was viewed as harsh and unpalatable. Thus, with the advent of diuretics in the 1950s, doctors largely switched from diet to drug therapy, which was effective and, they felt, was more practical.

Drugs of various kinds continued to be the major treatment modality for years until research raised a new concern. During the 1980s, studies indicated that it was important to treat mild hypertension (90–100 diastolic). By this criteria, 40 million people in the United States need treatment, although most of them don't need to lower their blood pressure by much. But more recent studies have raised concern about the fact that many of the drugs used to treat hypertension are associated with higher cholesterol levels. There is a significant question as to whether this rise in cholesterol may outweigh the good that antihypertensive drugs do for some people with mild hypertension. Consequently, dietary therapy has returned to the forefront as a major treatment for mild and moderate high blood pressure in people who have no other risk factors, and as an adjunct to drug therapy for everyone else with hypertension.

The 1988 report of the Joint National Committee on High Blood Pressure emphasizes weight reduction, salt restriction, and moderation of alcohol consumption as key to controlling blood pressure. And the report mentions increasing potassium and calcium intake, and lowering fat consumption, as additional factors. Thus, diet has been reinstated as a major treatment modality for all degrees of hypertension. Dietary intervention is particularly appropriate for a *take charge* approach. People have total control over their diet, and for almost everyone, dietary therapy has no negative side effects. Moreover, all the dietary recommendations for hypertension correspond to the Surgeon General's Report on national health recommendations for general good health, and will result in people feeling better and being less at risk of developing other illnesses, including heart disease, diabetes, and cancer.

NATIONAL HEALTH RECOMMENDATIONS AND DIETARY GOALS

1. Enough calories to meet body needs, but not more (fewer if overweight).
2. Less saturated fat, cholesterol.
3. Less salt.
4. Less sugar.
5. More whole grains, cereals.
6. More fruits and vegetables.
7. More fish, poultry.
8. More peas, beans.
9. Less red meat.
10. Avoid processed foods, or check ingredients carefully.

Source: The Surgeon General's Report *Healthy People,* 1980.

Diet, evolution, and taste

Due to a complex variety of factors, most people in Western industrialized countries do not eat a very healthy diet. In recent years, evolutionary biologists have theorized that our food cravings are the result of inborn bioprograms. Over many thousands of years, our bodies adapted to the food that we were able to obtain. Our primate ancestors ate a diet that consisted mainly of fruits and leaves, but as the brain of *homo sapiens* evolved and became larger and larger, humans needed a dramatic increase in calorie intake. Our brains use one-fifth of the calories we take in, and they need those calories all the time, not just while exercising. Early humans met their calorie needs with a diet of seeds, nuts, and meat—sources of calories which were infrequent, seasonal, and/or difficult to obtain. Anthropologists theorize that due to the relative scarcity of those high-calorie "packets" of energy, and the necessity of them for brain development, humans evolved to favor or seek out high-calorie, high-protein foods. Unfortunately for our health, this type of high-calorie, low-volume food is now readily available in industrialized countries, yet our inborn food cravings still remain high. This means that we now get too much of these foods too easily. Moreover, the fat that was found in

wild game was polyunsaturated, whereas the fat found in our do-
mesticated animals is highly saturated. Anthropologists have calcu-
lated that as compared to the average present-day Western diet,
hunter-gatherer peoples ate one-half the fat (which was more polyunsaturated), one-sixth the salt, twice the fiber, seven times the calcium, four times the vitamin C, and much more potassium; and, of
course, they had no refined sugar, flour, alcohol, or tobacco.

Catering to our inborn food preferences, the food and beverage
industries have produced and successfully advertised processed foods
that are high in salt, fat, and sugar, and low in nutrients. A graphic
example is the potato chip. The potato is similar to a tuber eaten by
hunter-gatherers, but the potato chip, its modern-day offspring, has six
times the calories, 400 times the fat, and 250 times the salt. Modern
advertising is remarkably persuasive, and processed foods are ubiqui-
tous. Since we are programmed by evolutionary needs to seek the
once-scarce foods that are high in protein, fat, salt, and sugar, and since
those foods are now so readily available in supermarkets and restau-
rants, we frequently eat a diet that is too high in calories, fat, salt, and
sugar. We have to make a *conscious decision* to eat a healthy diet.
Understanding the diet humans have evolved helps to explain why we
are attracted to certain types of food and find them so difficult to give

A HUNTER-GATHERER DIET AS COMPARED TO MODERN MAN'S

½ the fat (mostly polyunsaturated)

3 times as much protein

⅙ the salt

2 times the calcium

More potassium

4 times the vitamin C

2 times as much fiber

No refined sugar

No alcohol

No tobacco

DIET-RELATED DISEASES

Heart disease
High blood pressure
Non-insulin-dependent diabetes
Diverticulitis
Cancer of the colon
Irritable bowel syndrome
Cancer of the breast
Obesity

up. It should also make us feel less guilty about our cravings and occasional lapses.

Evidence that diet affects blood pressure

Researchers have found that a number of nutritional factors have an effect on the body's blood pressure, including sodium, potassium, calcium, magnesium, fiber, fat, obesity, a vegetarian diet, alcohol, and nicotine. Numerous studies have demonstrated that each of these factors by itself, has a small but definite effect on blood pressure. Taken as a group, their effects are significant. Rather than concentrate on just one ingredient, such as salt, it is far more effective to eat a healthy diet that encompasses all of these dietary factors. In one study, people with moderate hypertension were put on a high-fiber, low-fat, low-sodium diet. As compared to a control group, these people experienced a 10-point drop in diastolic blood pressure. One in three patients in the diet group was able to discontinue medication altogether; four out of five patients were able to stop or reduce their medication. It is also important to note that people in the study lost an average of five pounds, and reported feeling happier and less depressed.

Recent research has underscored the value of a nutritional approach to blood pressure control for millions of people who have mild hypertension, particularly in terms of heart disease. One study dealt with a group of men who were overweight and had mildly elevated blood pressure (154/96 without medication). These men were randomly as-

DIET AND HYPERTENSION

Diet approach	Average U.S. consumption	Levels used to treat hypertension	Comments
Sodium restricted	7–15 gms	Under 2 gms	Avoiding salty foods easily reduces intake to 3 gms. Effective for some, but not all, people.
Weight control	40 million overweight	Loss of 10–15 lbs.	Primary treatment for people who are overweight. Blood pressure decreases in relation to weight loss.
Alcohol restricted	Less than 2 oz. daily	No more than 1 oz./day	Effective treatment for people who are heavy drinkers.
Increased potassium	40–50 mEq	Greater than 80 mEq	May need supplements to achieve this level, which can cause stomach upset.
Increased calcium	400–600 mgs	Over 1,000 mgs	May need supplements to achieve this level.
Decreased fat	40–50% of caloric intake	10–25% of caloric intake	Reducing fat reduces heart disease risk by lowering cholesterol levels.
Increased fiber	7 gms/1000 calories	25 gms/1000 calories	Fiber supplements may be necessary to achieve this level.

signed to drug therapy (beta-blockers or diuretics) or to a low-calorie, low-sodium, low-fat, low-alcohol diet. At the end of one year, one-third of the patients on dietary therapy had lowered their blood pressure enough so that they definitely did not require any additional therapy, and many more had experienced a smaller drop in blood pressure and might not require additional therapy if they continued the diet. In general, people on the diet were able to reduce their intake of fat and calories, but were less successful with the other parts of the diet. Most interesting of all, the group treated with diet lowered their cholesterol by an average of 13 points and raised their levels of *HDLs (high-density lipoproteins),* the cholesterol fraction that helps to reduce the risk of heart disease. Among the men treated with drug therapy, two-thirds dropped their diastolic blood pressure below 90, but as a group, they showed a slight increase in their cholesterol levels and a drop in their HDL levels. For this population, an improvement in their lipid profile might be as important in preventing heart disease as lowering blood pressure. Thus the study concluded that it makes sense to use dietary therapy as the first line of treatment in people with mild, uncomplicated hypertension.

A research project with even broader implications dealt with *preventing* hypertension. The study involved people 30 to 44 years of age who had "high normal" blood pressure readings (85–89 mmHg diastolic), were slightly overweight, and/or had a slightly rapid pulse. Half the group was put on a low-calorie, low-salt, low-alcohol diet and assigned exercise. After five years, there was a 20% incidence of high blood pressure in the control group as compared with only an 8% incidence in the diet-and-exercise group. What is most interesting is that the measured changes between the two groups were actually very small: the diet group lost only an average of five pounds, and the control group actually showed a slight drop in their sodium and alcohol intake.

Weight reduction
There is a strong link between being overweight and having high blood pressure. Fat distribution seems to play a role. For unknown reasons, excess abdominal weight is more important than heaviness in the hips;

GUIDE FOR LOSING WEIGHT

1. Eat less total calories: in general, 100 extra calories a day over a long period gains 1 pound per month, 10 pounds per year.
2. Eat smaller portions; don't eat seconds.
3. Substitute low-calorie foods for high-calorie foods.
4. Rid the house of junk foods.
5. Have available low-calorie snacks such as carrots, celery, fruits, and unbuttered popcorn.
6. Avoid sugary or fatty desserts, such as cakes, pies, and ice cream.
7. Use non-fat dairy products instead of regular ones.
8. Remove fat from meat, skin from poultry.
9. Avoid fatty marbled meats such as duck, goose, frankfurters, sausage, hamburger.
10. Avoid butter, oil, shortening, lard, and fat.
11. Avoid fried foods, cream sauces, chocolate, alcohol, non-dairy creamers, and most packaged meals.
12. Keep an honest food record for one week.
13. Check the foods you eat against a calorie list.
14. Exercise at least 3 times a week; avoid long sedentary activities.

a large waistline is more likely to correlate with hypertension than a big hipline. Obesity affects all the factors that are associated with blood pressure, so that losing weight actually constitutes a multifaceted approach to treating hypertension. For many people, losing even 10–15 pounds is effective in lowering blood pressure.

Researchers have a good idea of the mechanics by which excess weight causes blood pressure to rise:

1) Obesity stimulates an increase in insulin production. This causes the kidney to absorb more sodium, which in turn causes greater water retention.

2) As weight and water retention go up, so does a person's blood volume. The greater the blood volume, the more blood the heart has to pump and the greater the cardiac output becomes.

3) Most people who are overweight not only eat more food, they consume more sodium as well, which increases their water retention and blood volume.

4) Obesity correlates with an increase in sympathetic nervous system activity, which is associated with a rise in blood pressure.

In a study of overweight people who had hypertension, it was found that 75% of those who lost 20 pounds or more achieved normal blood pressures through *weight loss alone*. This research has been corroborated by many similar studies. Nor did people's blood pressure go back up again once weight loss stopped. Interestingly, it has been found that weight reduction has a greater effect on lowering blood pressure if people are taken off antihypertensive drugs. Weight reduction also lessens the risk of heart attack by dropping the levels of cholesterol and LDLs (the fraction which transports cholesterol to the cells) while simultaneously raising the level of HDLs (the cardioprotective fraction). People who successfully lose weight report both cosmetic and physical benefits; they not only look better, they feel better. Thus weight loss is the first line of treatment in hypertensives who are overweight.

Sodium

Salt is essential for life—but in very *small* amounts. This need, coupled with the scarcity of salt in ancient times, caused early humans to evolve with a taste for salt, one of the most ancient condiments used in cooking. Salt is mentioned frequently in the Old Testament. In Roman times it was so scarce, and therefore so precious, that it was used as currency.

Salt consists of equal parts sodium and chloride (NaCl). It is the sodium in salt more than the chloride that is associated with hypertension. Sodium in foods comes from three sources. First, sodium occurs naturally in vegetables and meat because it is absorbed from soil and water. In the average American diet, this represents about 16% of overall sodium intake. In industrialized societies, 50% of sodium intake comes from processed foods, which are generally heavily flavored with salt. The other 34% of the sodium is applied by individuals using the salt shaker. In the U.S., women eat 2,000–4,000 mg of sodium per day, on the average, while men consume 4,000–6,000 mg per day

FACTS ABOUT SALT

1. The sodium in salt causes cells to retain water, which leads to high blood pressure in people who are salt sensitive.
2. Most Americans eat 4000 to 8000 mg of salt per day; for good health, the American Heart Association recommends only 2000 mg.
3. Under most conditions, people actually need only 250 mg of salt per day.
4. There's enough sodium in foods naturally to meet daily requirements without adding salt.

because they generally eat more. By comparison, hunter-gatherers are thought to have eaten 400–1,000 mg per day. It is estimated that to survive, people need only 250 mg per day. The average person today generally gets enough salt just from the vegetables and meat that he or she eats. Simply removing the salt shaker from the table does not

MINIMIZING SODIUM INTAKE

1. Don't add salt in cooking or at the table.
2. Use unprocessed foods which are naturally low in salt: grains and cereals, vegetables, fruits, fish, poultry, and meat.
3. Use non-fat dairy products that are lowest in salt: unsalted cottage cheese, non-fat cheese.
4. Eat fresh foods, which are naturally flavorful.
5. Avoid commercial salad dressings.
6. Use no-salt seasonings such as citrus fruits and juices, wine, dry mustard, parsley, garlic, onions, mushrooms, green peppers, apples, and other herbs and spices.
7. Avoid softened water, which is high in sodium.
8. Avoid over-the-counter and prescription drugs that contain sodium.

HIGH-SALT FOODS TO AVOID

Bouillon
Most packaged or canned soups
Meat tenderizers (salted)
Salted spices (e.g., garlic salt)
Soy and teriyaki sauce
Worcestershire sauce
Instant hot cereals
Instant chocolate drinks
Processed cheese, cheese products
American cheese
Cottage cheese
Parmesan cheese
Roquefort cheese
Salted crackers
Salted pretzels, chips, popcorn
Pickled foods
Olives
Sauerkraut
Vegetable juices
Bacon
Sausage
Frankfurters
Ham
Corned beef
Luncheon meats
Dried meat or fish
Salted, canned meat or fish
Most packaged or restaurant food

necessarily constitute a salt-restricted diet because most people consume a tremendous amount of salt in prepared foods. Although people complain that food is less palatable without salt, most find that they adjust to the lack of salt within a relatively short time, especially if they learn to season food with herbs and spices.

The implication that salt is a cause of high blood pressure initially came from research showing that cultures which eat a diet low in sodium have little or no hypertension. The success of the Kempner low-sodium, fruit-and-rice diet in treating hypertension verified these cross-cultural findings. Sodium raises blood pressure through a combined effect on several systems. First, it affects the kidneys' ability to excrete fluids, thereby raising the body's fluid volume. Second, sodium affects the sympathetic nervous system, making it more reactive and thus more responsive to norepinephrine, the hormone that controls the fight-or-flight reaction.

In spite of extensive studies linking sodium with hypertension, some researchers question how important a factor sodium is. Their reasoning is that a slight lowering of salt intake for a whole population with a high-salt diet does not have a great effect on the average blood pressure level. These researchers acknowledge a relationship between sodium and hypertension, but they feel it is too weak to recommend a restricted salt intake for an entire population, or even for everyone who has high blood pressure. Other researchers approach the data from the opposite vantage point. Pooled studies show an average decrease of 5–10 points diastolic, or more, in response to a low-salt diet. Many doctors feel that the drop in blood

CONVERSIONS BETWEEN SALT UNITS

Salt in grams	Sodium in milligrams	Sodium in milliequivalents
2.5 gm	1,000 mg	44 mEq
5	2,000	88
7.5	3,000	132
10	4,000	176

HIGH POTASSIUM FOODS

Oranges

Prunes

Bananas

Melons

Figs

Dates

Apricots

Raisins

Beans

Peas

Mushrooms

Potatoes

Spinach

Winter Squash

Sweet Potatoes

Tomatoes

pressure achieved through a low-salt diet is significant enough and valuable enough to recommend it for everyone with high blood pressure, and even as a general dietary guideline. This view is supported by the fact that salt restriction has no adverse effects in most people (in a small number of people, blood pressure actually rises when salt is restricted). The most recent large-scale study, the Intersalt Diet, which dealt with 10,000 men and women in 32 countries, did find a significant relationship between sodium and blood pressure.

Researchers now think that some people are sodium sensitive, that their blood pressure reacts to salt, unlike other people's. Sodium sensitivity is thought to be genetically determined and linked to low levels of renin, the kidney hormone that raises blood pressure. Unfortunately, no effective means has been devised to distinguish between those people who are salt sensitive and those who aren't. Despite the continued debate about sodium, most doctors feel that a low-salt diet is an effective part of any plan to lower blood pressure. In some cases the results of a low-salt diet will eliminate the need for medication entirely, in others it will reduce the dosage needed to lower blood pressure adequately.

Potassium

Many studies have shown an association between high potassium intake and low blood pressure, although the link has not been proven conclusively. Part of the problem in settling the question is that societies with a high-potassium diet tend to have a low sodium intake, and vice versa. It is therefore hard to determine whether low blood pressure averages are due to *high potassium* intake or to a *low sodium* intake. Among the studies that have tried to isolate the two factors, it has been found that higher potassium intake was associated with fewer strokes and lower blood pressure. Although the positive effects of potassium have not been totally proven, most doctors feel the evidence is convincing enough to recommend that people with high blood pressure increase their potassium intake since this has no side effects and is part of a healthy diet that prevents other diseases as well.

Natural sources of potassium are fruits and vegetables; the more of them people eat, the healthier their overall diet. These food sources are low-fat, low-cholesterol, and low-calorie, as well as low-sodium. Several studies have shown that taking potassium tablets as a dietary supplement causes a diastolic blood pressure drop of about 6 points after four weeks, but a number of other studies have not confirmed this. People on certain drugs (potassium-sparing diuretics or ACE inhibitors) should *not* take potassium supplements because their potassium levels are already high due to the drugs. However, since potassium-rich foods are part of a healthy diet, they are generally recommended as part of a total plan to lower blood pressure.

Calcium

In recent years, researchers have added calcium to the list of nutrients that are believed to affect blood pressure. Calcium plays an important role in heart contraction and normalizes sympathetic nervous system

HIGH-CALCIUM FOODS

Food	Amount	Calcium Content
Non-fat or low-fat milk	1 cup	350 mg
Non-fat or low-fat yogurt	1 cup	452 mg
Non-fat or low-fat cottage cheese	1 cup	211 mg
Oatmeal	¾ cup	188 mg
Salmon	3 oz.	170 mg
Broccoli	1 stalk	160 mg
Tofu	4 oz.	150 mg

Note: The daily calcium requirement is 800 mg for men, 1000 mg for premenopausal women, and 1400 mg for postmenopausal women.

activity. A group of studies showed that calcium supplementation (1 gm per day) caused an average drop in blood pressure of 4 points diastolic over a period of four weeks, while a four-year study showed that 1½ gms of calcium per day caused a drop of 10 points systolic. Not only does calcium supplementation have no side effects, it has other health benefits. These are particularly important in regard to osteoporosis, a disease in which bone density declines to the point that stress fractures become common. The disease largely affects postmenopausal women; as a group, they tend to have a low calcium intake.

Several epidemiological studies have shown that populations that eat a diet high in calcium tend to have low blood pressure. Conversely, other studies have shown that people with hypertension tend to eat a diet low in calcium. Studies also show that people with high blood pressure often metabolize calcium abnormally, causing them to have low blood levels of calcium. Still other studies show that there are lower death rates from heart disease in areas that have so-called "hard" water that contains calcium.

Fat and fatty acids

In recent years there has been a great deal of research into the effect of fat and fatty acids on blood pressure. Studies on both humans and animals have shown that a high-fat diet raises blood pressure, while a

GUIDE TO REDUCING DIETARY FAT/CHOLESTEROL

1. Use non-fat dairy products.
2. Use non-fat or skim-milk cheeses (ricotta, cottage, or farmer cheese).
3. Serve more poultry and fish, less red meat.
4. Trim all visible fat from meat.
5. Remove skin from poultry before cooking.
6. Use lean cuts of meat, not prime cuts.
7. Boil, bake, or steam meats and vegetables, rather than frying them.
8. Broil meat on racks to drain off fat.
9. Buy only fish that is canned in water.
10. Skim fat from soups, sautés.
11. Use oilless salad dressings.
12. Use non-fat yogurt and flavored vinegars in salad dressings.
13. Substitute non-fat yogurt for sour cream.
14. Substitute sorbet or non-fat ice cream.
15. Avoid using nuts and seeds.
16. Avoid high-fat luncheon meats and hot dogs.
17. Avoid or limit recipes using eggs.
18. Reduce egg yolks in recipes; replace with extra egg whites.
19. Avoid high fat crackers; check ingredients.
20. Avoid crackers, cookies, tortillas, etc., made with lard.
21. Substitute canola oil for lard or butter.
22. Substitute margarine for butter.
23. Avoid or limit use of shellfish.

---

* For a diet low enough in cholesterol to reverse existing heart disease, avoid meats and oils in addition.

diet generally low in fat tends to lower it. Some studies have even shown that simply replacing saturated fats with polyunsaturated fats—without even lowering the overall fat intake—resulted in a drop in blood pressure. It has been suggested by researchers that polyunsaturated fats are high in gamma linoleic acid which affects the synthesis of

TYPES OF FAT IN FOOD

Saturated fats*:	Monounsaturated fats*:
Butter	Avocado
Beef	Cashews
Veal	Olives
Pork	Olive oil
Poultry	Peanuts
Cheese	Peanut butter
Chocolate	Peanut oil
Coconut	**Polyunsaturated fats*:**
Coconut oil	Almonds
Egg yolk	Filberts
Lard	Pecans
Milk	Fish
Palm oil	Corn oil
Vegetable shortening (maybe)	Cottonseed oil
Ice Cream	Sunflower oil
Lobster	Safflower oil
Shellfish	Soybean oil
	Margarines**

* Saturated fats raise the level of cholesterol in the blood; monounsaturated and polyunsaturated fats do not.

** Margarines may contain saturated fat, depending upon what oils they are made from.

prostaglandins, potent substances that lower blood pressure by causing the arterioles to dilate.

Another area of research deals with the effect of polyunsaturated fish oils. Interestingly, these oils also lower cholesterol and improve inflammatory arthritis. Supplementation with both cod liver oil (5 ml per day) and commercial fish oil capsules (10–15 gms) has resulted in a slight lowering of blood pressure. Eicosapentaenoic acid, which is found in fish oils, is a component in prostaglandin synthesis. Although these studies do not include a large sample, they point to the fact that less saturated fat and the substitution of polyunsaturated fat will have a positive effect on blood pressure.

CHEESES THAT ARE HIGH IN FAT AND/OR SALT

Cheese	Fat content	Salt content
Low-fat processed cheese	Low	High
Low-fat creamed cottage cheese	Low	Very high
Camembert	Medium	High
Feta	Medium	High
Provolone	Medium	High
Romano	Medium	High
Processed American cheese food	Medium	High
Parmesan Cheese	Medium	Very high
Processed cheese spreads	Medium	Very high
Cream cheese	High	Low
Whole milk ricotta	High	Low
Cheddar	High	Medium
Monterey jack	High	Medium
Muenster	High	Medium
Processed American cheese	High	Very high
Blue cheese	High	Very high
Roquefort	High	Very high

Fiber

Because high fiber intake is characteristic of nonindustrialized societies that have a low incidence of hypertension, researchers have looked into whether high fiber intake, like low sodium consumption, contributes to low blood pressure values. Researchers were already aware that people on vegetarian diets have lower than average blood pressure, and vegetarian diets tend to be high in fiber. One study switched the eating habits of the participants so that those who normally ate a high-fiber diet were put on a low-fiber diet, and vice versa. Those people who increased their fiber experienced a drop in their blood pressure, while those who decreased their fiber showed a rise in blood pressure. Another study evaluated the difference between people who ate whole fruits and vegetables versus a group that consumed the same foods in juice form. Those who ate the foods as opposed to drinking the juices

CHOLESTEROL CONTENT OF FOODS

Food	Cholesterol in mg
Whole milk, 1c.	34
Skim milk, 1 c.	11
Cheddar cheese, 1 oz.	30
Ice cream, 1 c.	88
Egg, 1 whole	275
Butter, 1 T.	33
Margarine, 1 T.	0
Mayonnaise, 1 T.	10
Hot dog, 1	22
Lean red meat, ¼ lb.	80
Chicken, 100 gm	60
Fish, ¼ lb.	80
Lobster, ¼ lb.	225
Oysters, ¼ lb.	225
Shrimp, shelled, ¼ lb.	140
Lard, ¼ lb.	110

Note: The recommended daily allowance of cholesterol is 300 mg.

had lower blood pressures. Researchers estimate that a doubling of fiber in the average diet would drop blood pressure by 5%.

Since fiber, the skeletal remains of plants, is not even absorbed by the body, but simply passes through the digestive tract, the question arises as to how it can affect blood pressure. By adding bulk to the diet, fiber lowers the proportion of sugar and carbohydrates in a given meal, so the body makes less insulin in response. Since insulin causes sodium to be retained and results in an increase in fluid volume, lower insulin production tends to lower blood pressure. Although the correlation between fiber and hypertension is not very strong, a high-fiber diet has no negative side effects, is high in potassium, and plays a role in preventing other diseases such as gallstones, colon cancer, diabetes, and obesity.

CHOLESTEROL (mg/dl)

Risk	Total	LDL	Treatment
Recommended	<200	<130	Check on a regular basis.
Borderline	200-239	130-159	Without other risk factors, change diet and check annually; with risk factors, do aggressive diet and possibly drug therapy.
High	>240	>160	Make aggressive dietary changes and/or drug therapy.

[*] *Source:* National Cholesterol Education Program, 1988.

Vegetarian diets

Along with the renewed interest in dietary factors as they relate to blood pressure have come a group of studies on the effects of a vegetarian diet. Most vegetarian diets tend to be low in fat, and high in fiber and potassium. Many epidemiological studies comparing vegetarians and meat-eaters have shown vegetarians have lower average blood pressures. Although vegetarian diets involve a number of variables, and other lifestyle factors may play a role, studies that have attempted to balance for other factors still find that, on average, vegetarians have lower blood pressures. A number of research studies have found that putting people with hypertension on a vegetarian diet produced a lowering of diastolic blood pressure on the order of 5 points. Among a group of vegetarians who were willing to have meat added to their diet, researchers reported a rise in blood pressure, although this result could have been mediated by psychological factors. It is not surprising that a vegetarian diet decreases blood pressure because it involves a number of positive nutritional factors: vegetarian diets tend to be low in fat and sodium, and rich in fiber, potassium, and calcium.

DESIRABLE WEIGHTS FOR MEN AND WOMEN ACCORDING TO HEIGHT AND FRAME, AGES 25 AND OVER

Height (In Shoes)*	WEIGHT IN POUNDS (IN INDOOR CLOTHING)		
	Small Frame	Medium Frame	Large Frame
Men			
5'2"	112–120	118–129	126–141
3"	115–123	121–133	129–144
4"	118–126	124–136	132–148
5"	121–129	127–139	135–152
6"	124–133	130–143	138–156
7"	128–137	134–147	142–161
8"	132–141	138–152	147–166
9"	136–145	142–156	151–170
10"	140–150	146–160	155–174
11"	144–154	150–165	159–179
6'0"	148–158	154–170	165–184
1"	152–162	158–175	168–189
2"	156–167	162–180	173–194
3"	160–171	167–185	178–199
4"	164–175	172–190	182–204
Women			
4'10"	92–98	96–107	104–119
11"	94–101	98–110	106–122
5'0"	96–104	101–113	109–125
1"	99–107	104–116	112–128
2"	102–110	107–119	115–131
3"	105–113	110–122	118–134
4"	108–116	113–126	121–138
5"	111–119	116–130	125–142
6"	114–123	120–135	129–146
7"	118–127	124–139	133–150
8"	122–131	128–143	137–154
9"	126–135	132–147	141–158
10"	130–140	136–151	145–163
11"	134–144	140–155	149–168
6'0"	138–148	144–159	153–173

*1-inch heels for men and 2-inch heels for women.

NOTE: Prepared by the Metropolitan Life Insurance Company. Derived primarily from data of the *Build and Blood Pressure Study.*

DECREASING DIETARY SUGAR

---

1. Avoid cakes, candy, and cookies; instead, eat fresh fruits and low-sugar sorbets.
2. Avoid sugared soft drinks; substitute flavored mineral waters, or a combination of juice and seltzer water.
3. Avoid sugar in coffee or tea; substitute cinnamon or spices.
4. Use low-sugar jams.
5. Flavor pancakes with cinnamon, nutmeg, or vanilla extract.
6. Dilute pancake syrup with water.

Alcohol

Although the general public has not been much aware of it, doctors have long known that a high alcohol intake is associated with high blood pressure. As far back as 1915, alcoholism was demonstrated to be a cause of hypertension among French soldiers. In a recent study of 87,000 people in the Kaiser Health Plan, it was found that three or more drinks a day was a significant risk factor for hypertension. Another study showed that an intake of one ounce of alcohol per day was associated with a 2–6 point rise in diastolic pressure. The most recent studies show that the increase is linear, beginning with one or two drinks a day. Studies also show that blood pressure drops if drinking is stopped, but goes back up when drinking is resumed. Interestingly, in some alcoholics cessation of drinking will by itself bring blood pressure values back down to the normal range.

Researchers are not exactly sure how alcohol causes a rise in blood pressure, but animal studies show that alcohol intake is associated with a decrease in sodium excretion and an increase in blood volume. Animals who are fed alcohol also exhibit higher sympathetic nervous system activity. In addition, chronic stress is known to enhance alcohol's effect on raising blood pressure and stimulating the nervous system. It is important for people with hypertension to realize that alcohol often contributes to a rise in blood pressure, and they are advised to use alcohol infrequently and in small amounts.

HIGH-FIBER FOODS

Food	Fiber in gms
Bran or wheat germ, 1 T.	1
Whole wheat bread, 1 slice	2.7
White bread, 1 slice	0.8
Bran muffin, 1	3
Brown rice, ½ c.	1
High-fiber cracker, 1	2–3
Bran cereal, 1 oz.	4–13
Oatmeal, 1 oz.	2
Whole wheat spaghetti, 1 c.	4
Popcorn, 3 c.	2
Baked beans, ½ c.	9
Kidney beans, ½ c.	7
Lentils, ½ c.	4
Peas, ½ c.	4
Potato (with skin), 1	3.8
Sweet potato (with skin), 1	3
Zucchini, ½ c.	2.5
Broccoli, ½ c.	2
Tomatoes, ½ c.	2
Lettuce, 1 c.	1
Pear, 1	5
Blackberries, ½ c.	5
Apple, 1	4
Orange, 1	3
Prunes, 5	5
Banana, 1	2
Strawberries, ¾ c.	2.4
Psyllium seed, 1 t. (e.g., *Metamucil*)	3.4

Note: The recommended daily amount of fiber is 20–35 gms.

Hypertension and smoking

Although smoking is not strictly a dietary factor, it does represent something that people take into their bodies, and it does affect blood

SIGNS OF EXCESSIVE ALCOHOL USE

Symptoms:
Alcohol on breath
Flushed face
Irregular heartbeat
Rapid heartbeat
Night sweats
Black and blue marks
Cigarette burns
Gastrointestinal bleeding
Exaggerated reflexes

Laboratory findings:
Hypoglycemia
Low magnesium
Low chloride
Anemia
Elevated liver enzymes
Clotting deficiency
ECG abnormalities

Resulting diseases:
Cirrhosis of the liver
Gastritis
Gastrointestinal bleeding
Nerve disorders
Seizure disorders

pressure. Within minutes of smoking a cigarette there is a distinct rise in blood pressure, yet smokers don't have higher blood pressures in general. Smoking is, however, a major cardiovascular risk factor: it is associated with a much higher than average incidence of stroke, and more than twice the risk of coronary artery disease and death. Some researchers have postulated that almost *half* of all deaths from heart disease could be eliminated if everyone in the U.S. stopped smoking. It is interesting to note the people with hypertension who smoke do not

ALCOHOL CONTENT OF LIQUOR, WINE, AND BEER

Type	Alcohol (by percent)	Dose (in milliliters)	Dose (in ounces)	Alcohol content (in grams)	Alcohol calories (in kilo-calories)*
Liquor					
80 proof	40%	30 ml	1 oz.	12.0 gm	85 kcal
86 proof	43	30	1	12.9	92
90 proof	45	30	1	13.5	96
Wine					
Regular	10–12	120	4	13.2	93
Light	7–9	120	4	9.6	68
Beer					
Regular	4	360	12	14.4	153
Light	4	360	12	14.4	102

* Kilocalories from pure alcohol only, exclusive of carbohydrate content, etc.

respond as well to beta-blockers, one type of antihypertensive drug. Smokers who have high blood pressure are also more likely to develop *severe* hypertension. Finally, smoking is associated with higher than average levels of cholesterol and fibrinogen (a clotting agent), lower levels of protective HDLs, and abnormal platelet activity. Giving up smoking reverses most of these negative changes. A person's risk of stroke declines within two years and is comparable to that of a non-smoker within five years; the risk of coronary artery disease and death declines within five years, and is similar to that of nonsmokers within ten years.

Taking charge of your diet
The first step in taking charge of your diet is to understand what dietary factors are known to affect hypertension. That has been the goal of the first part of this chapter. To summarize, studies have shown

GIVING UP SMOKING

If you are thinking about quitting:

1. Think of what you will gain by quitting: time, money, better health, increased longevity, general sense of well-being, improved physical condition for exercise, personal sense of being in control, respect of others.
2. Realize that by quitting you will make others healthier and set a good example, especially for your children.
3. Make a list of all the reasons why you want to quit.
4. Set a firm target date for quitting.
5. Try to get someone else to be a "buddy" and quit with you.
6. Make a contract with someone about your quitting; have that person support you, monitor you.

Ways to cut down before quitting totally:

1. Switch to a different brand that is low in tar and nicotine, or is just distasteful.
2. Smoke only half of each cigarette.
3. Limit smoking by number or hour: postpone the first cigarette of the day, smoke only a set number of cigarettes per hour, etc.
4. Don't keep extra cigarettes around; purchase them by the pack.
5. Stop carrying cigarettes; keep them in a place that is hard to get at.
6. Stop smoking at home, at work, in public places, or in the car.
7. Reach for gum, low-calorie foods, or water when you want a cigarette.
8. Don't clean your ashtrays; alternatively, keep all your cigarette butts in a large glass jar.

When you actually stop smoking:

1. Rid the house and car of all cigarettes, butts, ashtrays, lighters, and matches.
2. Make a list of what you can buy with the money you save daily, weekly, or monthly.
3. Keep busy.
4. Exercise frequently.
5. Buy something to keep your hands busy, such as paper clips, pencils, wind-up toys, or begin new projects like knitting or needlepoint.
6. Drink large quantities of water, seltzer, and fruit juice.
7. When you'd usually smoke, get up and walk or do something else.
8. Avoid places where people are smoking.
9. Temporarily avoid situations and people that you associate with smoking.
10. Increase activities where you can't smoke, such as exercising, going to the movies, etc.
11. Do relaxation exercises to relieve tension.

GIVING UP SMOKING (cont.)

12. Use imagery exercises to strengthen your motivation and get your mind off smoking.

13. Mark your progress—celebrate when you've been free of cigarettes for 1 day, 1 week, 1 month, and so on.

14. Never think you can smoke just 1 cigarette—you're almost certain to start smoking again.

15. If you're thinking of having a cigarette, call a friend whom you've set up as a support person.

CONDITIONS ASSOCIATED WITH SMOKING

Lung cancer
Emphysema
Bronchitis
Colds
Heart attacks
Angina
Strokes
Peptic ulcers
Cancer of the larynx, mouth, esophagus, bladder, pancreas
Miscarriage
Low-birth-weight babies
Asthma

that a combined approach that involves losing weight (if necessary); lowering sodium, saturated fat, and alcohol consumption; and increasing potassium, calcium, and fiber intake will have the maximum effect on bringing blood pressure down. Any one of these interventions will have some effect, but the combination of several will produce even better results. Probably the most important among these interventions are weight loss and sodium restriction. Although it does not have a direct effect on lowering blood pressure, reducing cholesterol intake is also crucial because cholesterol is a major risk factor for heart attack, which accounts for the greatest number of deaths among people with hypertension.

Once you know what factors are important in your diet, the next

BENEFITS OF QUITTING SMOKING

1. More energy.
2. Less fatigue.
3. More stamina for exercise.
4. Greater sense of taste.
5. Better sense of smell.
6. Cleaner teeth.
7. No more stale cigarette odor on body, clothes.
8. Fewer colds.
9. More money.
10. Greater sense of self-control.
11. Increased pride.
12. Less fear of cancer, heart disease.

step is to *honestly* assess what you eat. The most effective way is to keep a record for one week of your daily intake of foods, beverages, and seasonings, including all between-meal snacks. It is very important to keep track of quantities and portion size—one cracker is far different from six. It is also very enlightening to briefly record the time and place at which you ate, how fast you ate, and what your mood was. Evaluating a week's record will help you determine what changes are needed in your diet with regard to calories, fat, cholesterol, sodium, potassium, calcium, alcohol and/or fiber. Try to get an objective idea of those nutritional factors on which you are above or below the recommendations for a healthy diet. Your ideal weight can be determined from the included table. Even being 5–10 pounds overweight can be significant in terms of hypertension.

People's food habits and addictions are complexly intertwined with their view of themselves, their upbringing, the stress they feel, and the support they receive from their family and friends. In other words, food habits are deeply tied to a person's psychological state and are often resistant to change. For all but a few people, the process is not simply a matter of rationally reviewing nutritional information and matter-of-factly instituting dietary changes. Many hypertension clinics and some holistic cardiologists address these problems directly through nutritional counseling. Any doctor who does not provide such counseling will be able to refer patients who request help. Groups such as Weight Watchers can also be of great benefit for those whose weight is a primary issue. Some people find that a close observation of their food habits and preferences brings up psychological issues that may best be dealt with through psychological counseling. This is particularly true for people who are severely overweight and are repeatedly unsuccessful with dieting.

Every person with high blood pressure is unique, but a majority are at least slightly overweight and can do much to improve their diet in terms of hypertension. Depending on their customary diet, people will find that some nutritional issues are more important to deal with than others. Also, different people will find different interventions easier to make. Ultimately, these changes need to be lifetime changes. Some people can make sweeping changes all at once, while others do best by making changes gradually or dealing with one nutritional factor at a time.

Based on knowledge of how nutritional factors affect hypertension, and a careful assessment of their diet, people can go on to the next step—making a decision to change their diet and setting reasonable goals. There are three basic strategies for dietary change: *eliminating* (or *restricting*) unhealthy foods, *substituting* healthy foods for ones that are unhealthy, and *reducing* portion size. Thus, people who are overweight might decide that their meals are relatively healthy, but that their portion sizes are too large, that they eat too much high-calorie food between meals, and that they should be more moderate in their salt consumption. Another person's goal might be to cut out between-meal snacks and lower salt consumption initially and to work on portion sizes at a later time. The point is to begin making changes and to make steady progress over a period of weeks and months.

Once people set their goals and begin to make changes, they often encounter problems with sticking to their goals. Motivation psychologists have identified a number of such "barriers to adherence":

1) *Lack of motivation:* the person expects a nutritionist or family member to do it for them.

2) *Excessive social pressure:* a person's job or family requires eating out much of the time.

3) *Lack of support:* family members aren't supportive and don't want their own diet to be changed.

4) *Emotional or self-regulatory problems:* a person sets up impossible goals or deadlines, and then gives up when these goals can't be met. Or the person is driven to eat enormous quantities of food, often out of loneliness, despair, boredom, or stress. People with these types of problems often experience cravings and eat large quantities of foods such as ice cream, cookies, or granola.

5) *Food preparation problems:* people who do not like to shop or prepare foods, or don't plan well, end up eating processed or prepared foods that are generally high in salt and fat.

Once people improve their diet, the goal becomes to maintain the new habits. One of the major long-term problems people encounter is that if they have a brief lapse or slip, they simply give up on all the changes they've made and return to their former eating habits. People need to realize that lapses are common, and will not have a major effect if their new food patterns are directly resumed. People are more likely to overcome brief lapses if they believe their blood pressure can be controlled, and if they are getting encouragement and positive feedback from their family, their doctor, or a support group. A positive attitude is crucial to the success of all dietary interventions. That is why it is so important for people to set their own goals, monitor their own blood pressure, and feel free to work on those nutritional areas they are most interested in. In time, the feelings of control and success that come from maintaining effective dietary interventions will improve people's attitude toward solving other problems in their life.

CHAPTER FIVE

Hypertension and Exercise

Physical exercise has a significant effect on blood pressure. Several major studies have shown that active people have an average diastolic blood pressure 2–5 points lower than nonactive people. A study on Harvard alumni found that people who did not exercise were 35 percent more likely to develop high blood pressure than those who did exercise. Other studies have shown that if exercise is done at least three times a week for 30-minute sessions, blood pressure drops an average of 6 points diastolic and 11 points systolic. The most effective type of exercise program is aerobic and involves rhythmic movement of large muscle groups. Examples are brisk walking, jogging, bicycling, cross-country skiing, swimming, aerobic workouts, or working with aerobic machines. Weight lifting and isometric exercises (contracting a muscle with no movement) are *not* recommended for anyone with hypertension. They have not been shown to lower blood pressure in the long run, and they can actually raise blood pressure markedly during workouts.

Regular exercise should be a part of any program to take charge of your blood pressure. In fact, the 1988 Report of the Joint Committee on Hypertension recommended that exercise be included as part of any nondrug therapy for mild hypertension, and as an adjunct to drug therapy for moderate-to-severe hypertension. Because hypertension is a risk factor for cardiovascular disease, doctors generally recommend that people with high blood pressure have a physical exam and possibly a stress test before initiating a serious exercise program.

BENEFITS OF REGULAR AEROBIC EXERCISE

1. Increased lung capacity.
2. Lower breathing rate.
3. Lower heart rate at rest.
4. Lower heart rate during exercise.
5. Increased blood volume per heartbeat.
6. Lower blood pressure.
7. Lower LDL cholesterol levels.
8. Higher HDL cholesterol levels.
9. Lower triglyceride levels.
10. Lower uric acid levels.
11. Decreased platelet stickiness.
12. Increased muscle strength.
13. Increased flexibility.
14. Increased physical skill.
15. Increased muscle capacity.
16. Increased insulin receptor sensitivity.
17. Increased sense of physical well-being.
18. Increased sense of mental well-being.
19. Reduced depression and anxiety.

During exercise, blood pressure rises sharply in order to supply more blood to working muscles. This is true for nonhypertensives as well as for people with high blood pressure. The rise is the same in both groups, but the peak levels reached are much higher in people with hypertension. Although this rise is not dangerous in people with normal blood pressure or *mild* hypertension, aerobic exercise should not be attempted by people with *untreated* moderate-to-severe hypertension because exercise can make their systolic blood pressure go up by as much as 40 points. Most doctors would say that a vigorous exercise program should not be initiated if blood pressure is above 175/110. Once blood pressures above this level are adequately reduced with medication, an exercise program can be started.

Exercise habits and human evolution

Everybody feels better when they exercise. Exercise helps people to build muscle tone, lose weight, increase their energy, and improve their mental outlook. Exercise is considered natural in childhood, but as people grow older, they tend to build their work and leisure habits around activities that are sedentary, and become more and more pre-occupied with the nonphysical aspects of their life. By middle age, people all too often find themselves somewhat overweight, with poor muscle tone, limited flexibility, and little aerobic capacity. When people are in this shape, the good feelings that exercise engenders are a dim memory. Once people get used to feeling somewhat achy, sluggish, and stiff, they find it hard to believe that they can feel otherwise, and incorrectly ascribe good physical feelings to youth. To undertake an exercise program, they have to alter their habits and be convinced that they can actually be physically active again. To accomplish such a change requires a conscious commitment to exercise regularly three times a week in order to get in shape.

Throughout most of mankind's evolution, human beings were phys-ically active for the whole of their lifetimes. In fact, the skeletons of our Paleolithic ancestors are comparable to those of well-conditioned ath-letes of the present. Based on skeletal comparisons, the average person today is only one-third as fit as our early ancestors. The fitness of Paleolithic peoples was not "planned," it was simply part of their lifestyle, which involved gathering fruits and vegetables, and hunting for game. For hunter-gatherer peoples, exercise was continuous, var-ied, and necessary; it simultaneously involved both strength and en-durance training. Given the evolutionary requirements that our bodies evolved for, it is not surprising that lack of exercise plays a part in many of our modern-day illnesses. Frequent, vigorous exercise has been found to reduce the risk of heart disease, diabetes, osteoporosis, and depression, as well as high blood pressure.

The physiology of how exercise causes a drop in blood pressure

Over a period of time, exercise lowers blood pressure by causing the arterioles to dilate, which in turn lessens vascular resistance to blood

CONDITIONS IMPROVED BY EXERCISE

Heart disease
High blood pressure
Non-insulin-dependent diabetes
Osteoporosis
Arthritis
Low back pain
Obstructive lung disease

flow. Exercise also decreases sympathetic nervous system activity, and probably lowers renin activity in the kidneys, both of which lessen constriction of the arterioles.

Exercise training produces significant physical changes by gradually requiring the body to supply greater and greater amounts of blood to the voluntary muscles. The amount of blood that a person's heart pumps out to the body depends almost completely on the amount of work or exercise that person *usually* does. The heart and the blood vessels in the muscles adapt to whatever level of work is required of them. When work increases steadily over a period of weeks or months, the size of the muscle fibers increases, the blood supply to the muscles increases, and most importantly, the heartbeat becomes more powerful so that more blood is pumped out with each beat. In effect, the heart pumps more and more efficiently, and even the mitochondria, the microscopic energy factories in the cells, become more efficient. This means that under any workload the heart has to pump fewer times to accomplish the same amount.

The autonomic nervous system, the part of the nervous system that maintains automatic functions such as heartbeat and breathing, also becomes more efficient with regular exercise. After exertion or stress, the system is quicker to drop back to a resting state and stay there. This toning of the autonomic nervous system works in situations of both emotional and physical stress. In sedentary people and people who are under emotional stress, the autonomic nervous system tends to remain in a slightly aroused state which causes the heart to beat faster and blood pressure to remain slightly elevated. In a person who does regular physical exercise, both the heartbeat and the blood pressure tend to reach a lower resting value. In fact, as a result of training, athletes have a lower-than-average resting pulse. This is not only due to the fact that their hearts pump more with each beat (increased cardiac output), but also to the fact that their sympathetic nervous system is less active. The main reason that blood pressure decreases in response to training is that the resistance of the arteries drops markedly. This occurs because during exercise the arterioles dilate to a greater extent in order to deliver more blood to the voluntary muscles. Studies have shown a 15–22% reduction in vascular resistance in response to training three to seven times a week.

The studies on exercise reducing blood pressure show excellent results. Over 25 controlled studies have been done in the last several years, using men and women between the ages of 20 and 70. The exercise groups engaged in aerobic exercise such as biking, running, walking, or calisthenics three times a week for 30 to 120 minutes per session. The training programs produced average increases in exercise capacity of 6–40%. Taken as a group, the studies demonstrated a drop of 11 points systolic and 6 points diastolic in people with high blood pressure. Interestingly, people who were not hypertensive did not demonstrate this drop in blood pressure. Two studies that employed continuous 24-hour blood pressure monitoring showed that among hypertensive people who participated in an exercise program, their blood pressure dropped during the day when it had usually been high, but did not drop at night when it was usually lower.

Setting up a personal exercise program

Studies have shown that in order to get optimum blood pressure reduction from an exercise program, vigorous aerobic exercise should be done at least three times a week for 30 minutes or more at a time. Vigorous aerobic exercise is defined as large muscle movement that makes an increased demand on the heart to pump blood out to the large muscles. During aerobic exercise, the stress load should reach at least 50% of a person's maximum ability to bring oxygen to the muscles. Such a demand is reflected in a rise in pulse rate during exercise.

The *pulse rate*, the number of times the heart beats per minute, is a

TARGET PULSE RATES FOR EXERCISE

- *Maximum heart rate* is determined by subtracting your age from 220.
- 45–80% of a person's maximum heart rate is the *target* for most effective aerobic training.
- Check pulse immediately upon ceasing exercise. Because pulse rate normally drops very quickly, count pulse for only ten seconds, then multiply by 6 to determine rate.
- Dr. Kenneth Cooper's formula for maximum heart rate for people on beta-blockers (e.g., Inderal) is 195 minus 80% of age minus 20% of drug dosage. For example, a 40-year-old on 50 mg of Inderal would use a maximum heart rate of $195 - (.80 \times 40 = 32) - (.20 \times 50 = 10) = 153$.

good measure of how much blood the heart is putting out. Since the pulse drops quickly as soon as a person stops exercising, the rate is determined most accurately by counting the pulse for 10 seconds and multiplying that figure by six. For a healthy person, the maximum ability to supply oxygen to the muscles corresponds to a pulse of 220 minus the person's age. People who are on beta-blockers cannot raise their heart rate this far, and should use a different formula (see chart).

People with diagnosed high blood pressure who have not been exercising regularly should consult their doctor before undertaking vigorous exercise. Generally, a physical exam and possibly a stress test are recommended since hypertension is a risk factor for cardiovascular disease. A stress test can pick up signs of blockage in the coronary arteries, which would limit the intensity of exercise that a person should engage in. A stress test will also help the doctor determine what training rate a person should initially set as a goal.

People who are out of shape or who are exercise beginners should not try to reach their training-goal rate immediately. Training physiologists advise people to start with a maximum pulse rate of 110, and build up to their goal level over a period of weeks. In addition, people who are just beginning a program should not exercise for 30 minutes straight if it makes them very tired. And people should *never* exercise to the point of exhaustion or strain. Often people begin an exercise program so enthusiastically that they do not pay close attention to their body's signals. It's important to realize that beginning to exercise can cause strain or exhaustion if people start out too fast or do too much at the beginning. This can not only be dangerous, it sometimes produces such discomfort that people stop exercising altogether. In terms of their heart, there are two simple signs that people are overdoing their exercise: (1) during exercise, they develop tightness in their chest, shortness of breath, lightheadedness, or muscle pain; (2) within 5–10 minutes after ending exercise, they still feel breathless and/or their heart rate has not dropped significantly.

Exercise physiologists have several tips for helping people plan a personal program that will be the most beneficial and the least dangerous. First, they emphasize strongly the value of *warming up* before beginning to exercise, and *cooling down* after exercise. They advise 5 minutes of stretching before beginning exercise to minimize joint or muscle injury. After exercising, they recommend 5 minutes of slow walking to return blood from the exercising muscles to other parts of the body. Without a cool-down period, people can become dizzy. In general, people should exercise at the same time each day so as to make it a habit. Exercising at lunchtime is especially valuable for people who are overweight since it shortens the time for them to eat.

The most important thing for beginners is to start their program *very gradually,* over a period of 6 weeks. Exercise physiologist Dr. Kenneth Cooper suggests, for example, that in the first week people between 40 and 50 years of age who are out of shape simply attempt to walk one mile in about 20 minutes. As they feel comfortable, they can gradually increase both their speed and distance. At the end of 6 weeks, the goal would be to do about 2 miles in 30 minutes. By the end of 16 weeks, when the people feel they are in good condition, the goal would be to walk 4 miles in about 45–60 minutes.

Special exercise advice is necessary for people on beta-blockers. These drugs limit heart rate significantly enough to affect training. At the Institute for Aerobics Research, Dr. Cooper has found that people who are on beta-blockers benefit from exercise, but they should not try

CALORIES EXPENDED BY EXERCISE

Type of exercise	Calories consumed per hour
Sleeping	80
Sitting	100
Standing	140
Driving	120
Light housework	180
Walking (slow: 2.5 mph)	210
Biking (slow: 5 mph)	210
Gardening	220
Golf	250
Mowing with a power mower	250
Bowling	270
Swimming (slow: 1/4 mph)	300
Walking (brisk: 3.75 mph)	300
Horseback riding	350
Volleyball	350
Ping-Pong	360
Tennis	420
Hill climbing	480
Swimming (moderate: 2 mph)	500
Racquetball	600
Biking (fast: 13 mph)	660
Running (moderate: 10 mph)	900

to reach the same maximum heart rate as people with other treatment regimens. This will not affect individuals doing average aerobic exercise, but it probably would affect an athlete with a very vigorous exercise program. People on beta-blockers will still increase their aerobic fitness, and will experience the beneficial effect on their blood pressure. Those people who find that beta-blockers impair their physical exercise program should consult with their doctor about switching to other hypertensive medications.

ADVICE FOR EXERCISING SAFELY

1. Get in shape slowly.
2. Before exercising, warm up for 5–10 minutes by doing stretches, sit-ups, or slow movement.
3. Exercise regularly: 3–5 times per week, 20–30 minutes per session, at a pulse rate that is 45–80% of maximum (220 minus your age). People on beta-blockers should use the formula on page 100.
4. After exercising, cool down for 5–10 minutes by doing slowdown activities or stretches.
5. Stop exercising if you experience fatigue, breathlessness, or pain.

SUGGESTIONS FOR INCREASING DAILY ACTIVITY LEVEL

1. Stand instead of sitting or reclining.
2. Whenever possible, walk instead of driving.
3. Park or get off bus several blocks from your destination; walk between stores.
4. Use stairs instead of elevators or escalators.
5. Do your own housecleaning and yard work.
6. Take short walks during work breaks.
7. Walk with your dog.
8. Walk and talk with friends, instead of sitting and talking.

The long-term goal of any exercise program is to maintain it. The first month or so is the hardest. Not only is your body getting used to exercise, you are trying to cultivate a new habit. During this period people do not fully experience the invigorating, even addictive, effects of exercise. Exercise physiologists generally report that people are most likely to be successful in undertaking an exercise program if they make a decision to do it for at least 8 weeks. During that time, it's important to reward yourself and get support from others to help you stick with it. The exercise habit will not yet be ingrained, and your natural resistance will be greatest at this time. Also, as we said, people tend to get carried away in the beginning, often injuring or straining themselves, and end up never actually exercising on a steady basis. Finally, when you commit to exercising for 8 weeks, it's important to pick the type of exercise that you feel you'd enjoy the most, that would be best for you (taking into account any other medical conditions), and that you'd be most able to accommodate in your daily schedule. The more carefully you choose your exercise in terms of pleasure, scheduling, and your general health, the more likely you are to make it a part of your life.

CHAPTER SIX

Hypertension Drugs

Extensive research has documented that lowering high blood pressure reduces the incidence of illness and death from strokes and heart attacks in people with moderate and severe hypertension (greater than 104 diastolic). In patients with mild hypertension (90–104 diastolic), studies show that blood pressure reduction lowers the risk of stroke by 30–50%, but it has not been shown to be protective against heart attack, probably because heart disease is affected by a number of factors, including cholesterol level and smoking habits. In recent years, lifestyle changes (diet, exercise, stress reduction) have been the initial treatment of choice for people with mild high blood pressure, and even for some people with moderate hypertension and no other risk factors for heart disease. However, drug therapy remains the mainstay of treatment for moderate and severe high blood pressure, and even for mild high blood pressure if there are other risk factors involved.

Recently, a number of new hypertension drugs have been developed that make treating high blood pressure easier, and that have fewer side effects than older drugs. Using these medications, most hypertensive patients can reduce their blood pressure to a normal level (140/90 mmHg) without any other changes in their lifestyle. The success of these drugs has taken a great deal of the danger out of moderate and severe hypertension, a fact that should be very reassuring for people whose diastolic pressure is over 105.

Hypertension involves a complex group of changes in the body's physiology. Because they don't have any symptoms, many people with high blood pressure object to having to take drugs "as if they were sick." Others feel they should be able to control their blood pressure consciously, and are unhappy when they cannot. Because so many factors affect blood pressure, most people with moderate-to-severe hypertension cannot control their blood pressure without the help of medication. Through lifestyle changes many people in the moderate-to-severe range have been able to achieve enough of a reduction in blood pressure to lower their medication, but not that many have been successful in eliminating their need for medication entirely. With more assertive lifestyle changes, and perhaps with the help of nutritionists, counselors, or hypnotherapists, highly motivated people may be able to achieve and maintain even greater reductions in blood pressure. But if that is not possible, people should not feel badly about using medication as a helper. They have not done something wrong, and they have not failed. Nor should people feel that they are "ill" in the sense of being handicapped. By taking medication if they need it, they are protecting their health and enhancing the quality of their life.

From a medical point of view, the major problem with antihypertensive drugs is the fact that a significant percentage of people don't take their medication regularly or stop taking it altogether. Doctors often tend to blame patients for this, and label it "noncompliance," without really looking into the reasons for it. Studies indicate the main problem is that people often do not really understand why they are taking the drugs, and they do not feel involved in or responsible for their treatment. Since people don't have symptoms alleviated by the drugs, they have little motivation to take medication daily. Moreover, some people resent having to take a drug because that implies that they are "sick," and they do not think of themselves as sick. Finally, some antihypertensive drugs do produce side effects in a percentage of the people who take them. We will discuss these side effects and what can be done about them under the specific types of drugs. Mutual participation on the part of doctor and patient is needed, and people have to understand that taking medication is a crucial part of their participation in effective treatment of their hypertension.

The goals of antihypertensive medications

The basic goal of antihypertensive drug therapy is to lower people's blood pressure to normal levels with as few drugs as possible, using as low a dosage as possible, and with as few side effects as possible. Ideally, people can be maintained on one drug, at a low dose, with minimal or no side effects. In the past twenty-five years, four different types of antihypertensive medications, with different physiological modes of action, have been used in the initial treatment of hypertension. Each of the drugs, by itself, has been found to lower blood pressure to normal levels in approximately half the people treated. Different people respond better to one type of drug or another, depending upon which factors play the most important role in their hypertension. Unfortunately, it is difficult or impractical for a doctor in clinical practice to determine the major underlying mechanism. In fact, in most cases no one mechanism predominates.

Arriving at the "best" drug regimen is, to some degree, a matter of trial and error based on the doctor's knowledge of the drugs and the patient's response to them. Doctors use a complex set of generalizations in determining which type of drug to prescribe initially. These generalizations involve age, sex, race, physical exam findings, lab values, associated illnesses and risk factors. They are useful because certain physiological mechanisms are more common in young people as compared to older people, in one race as compared to another, and in men as compared to women. For example, older people and blacks are more likely to have hypertension caused by increased blood volume in association with a low renin output, whereas younger people and whites are more likely to have hypertension caused by a high renin output. Based on all of a person's characteristics, the doctor will choose the class of drug he or she believes will be most effective. Making this choice is an art as much as a science, and the doctor's first choice sometimes does not lower the blood pressure sufficiently, or occasionally side effects make the drug undesirable from the patient's point of view. In either of these cases, the doctor will change the dose or switch to another type of drug after several weeks. This does not mean that either the doctor or the patient has "failed," it just means the drug did not match the patient's physiology as well as it could.

For the past twenty years, the treatment regimen for hypertension has been referred to as *stepped care*. Initially people were put on diuretics, and then other drugs were added if their blood pressure did not come down sufficiently. People whose blood pressure was not responsive might be put on several drugs. Whereas diuretics had been widely used, the other drugs were newer and had not been used as extensively. Eventually, several problems caused doctors to reappraise the stepped-care approach. First, the stepped-care regimen did not take into account individual differences. Second, by the mid-1980s studies had also shown that diuretics caused cholesterol levels to rise, which, particularly in people with mild high blood pressure, might be as serious a risk factor as their hypertension. Meanwhile, new drugs had become available that had different modes of action, but were also suitable as initial therapy. Doctors realized that in some cases it would be preferable to use an agent with a different mechanism rather than follow the old regimen of adding one drug to another.

The current approach, which is called *individualized step-care,* involves starting a person on one of the four main classes of antihypertensive drugs: *diuretics, beta-blockers, calcium antagonists,* or *ACE (angiotensin-converting enzyme) inhibitors.* The choice of which type of drug to use initially is based on the person's individual characteristics and risk factors. If the first drug does not produce an adequate drop in blood pressure, there are three options, again depending on the person's individual makeup. One option is to increase the dose of the initial drug; another is to add a second drug with a different mechanism; and the third is to stop the initial drug and substitute one with a different mechanism. In general, a combination of drugs allows the doctor to prescribe low dosages, which tends to minimize side effects. If the second drug or drug combination is also ineffective, other substitutions or combinations will be tried in sequence. If one of the four basic classes of drugs is not successful, there are other antihypertensives that are sometimes used in combination with the basic ones.

In addition to a more individualized approach to the choice of antihypertensive drugs, there is also a new philosophy that considers *step-down,* that is reducing dosages or withdrawing medication for a trial period. This approach is tried after people have successfully controlled their blood pressure with medication for a year, particularly in cases of mild high blood pressure. Doctors are finding that it is often possible for people to step down, especially if they have undertaken effective lifestyle changes.

It is important for people to realize that there are many more options in drug therapy than there used to be, and that doctors are taking a much more individualized approach to therapy. Often the best treatment involves trying several different regimens to arrive at the ideal approach. With individualized step-care, it's very important that people communicate to their doctor how they feel and whether they have an objectionable side effects. Given the large number of antihypertensive drugs and the new flexibility in treatment, people should be able to work successfully with their doctor to find a regimen that they are comfortable with and can maintain.

Diuretics

Diuretics, the oldest and best-known blood pressure medication, are still the most widely used. Basically, *diuretics* cause the kidneys to excrete more salt and more water, thereby lowering the body's blood volume. As we've said, when blood volume is decreased, the heart has to pump less, and therefore cardiac output goes down. In addition to lowering cardiac output, diuretics also reduce peripheral vascular resistance. Researchers believe that this decline is caused by changes in the fluid content of the cells in the blood vessel walls. Diuretics are prescribed alone and in combination with other drugs. They work especially well in older people, people who are overweight, blacks, and people who have increased blood volume with low renin activity.

The adverse effects of diuretics are due to the metabolic changes that they cause. These include a drop in potassium and magnesium levels, and a rise in glucose, uric acid, cholesterol and serum lipids. A decrease in potassium can cause fatigue, muscle weakness and cramps, and palpitations. These can be offset by a diet rich in potassium, by potassium supplements, or by potassium-sparing agents. In the case of people who are diabetic, the rise in glucose may require adjustments in their insulin dosage. Among those people who are genetically susceptible to gout, the increase in uric acid can precipitate an attack involving the sudden, painful inflammation of a joint. In some people, the most serious, long-term adverse effect is an increase in cholesterol and serum lipids, both of which are risk factors for heart disease. Adverse effects vary depending upon the person and the dosage prescribed. All of these factors, especially the rise in cholesterol, are causing doctors to use diuretics less commonly as initial drugs in the treatment of hypertension.

In addition to the metabolic changes they cause, diuretics can produce several side effects. These definitely do *not* occur in everyone, and are somewhat dosage dependent. By listing them here we do not mean to suggest that people are likely to experience them. Most people do not get side effects from these commonly used medications. Like other blood pressure medications, diuretics can cause lightheadedness with sudden changes in position. People who notice this effect can avoid it by getting up more gradually. Diuretics can also cause a tendency toward dehydration, which may be noticeable in extreme heat, after heavy exercise, or with diarrhea and vomiting. In any of these situations, people should make a point to drink more fluids than normal. In men, diuretics can cause the inability to maintain an erection, a condition which disappears when the drug is changed or the dosage is lowered. In both men and women, diuretics sometimes cause sun sensitivity and produce a rash when people go in the sun.

Beta-adrenergic receptor blocking agents, or beta-blockers

Beta-adrenergic receptor blocking agents, commonly known as *beta-blockers,* are a class of antihypertensive medication that lower blood pressure by preventing nerve impulses from reaching muscle cells. The sympathetic nervous system raises blood pressure in two ways—by stimulating the heart to beat faster and harder, and by causing the smooth muscle cells in the blood vessels to contract. The sympathetic nerves do not stimulate the muscle tissue directly, rather they release a chemical, *norepinephrine,* which is picked up by *beta receptors* on the surface of the muscle tissue. Beta-blocking drugs bind onto these receptors continuously, preventing norepinephrine from attaching to the sites and raising blood pressure. Beta-blockers reduce the rate and force of the heartbeat, thereby lowering cardiac output, and they also lower renin release from the kidney. Because beta-blockers lessen the work of the heart, they are particularly valuable for people who have existing heart disease, including people who have had previous heart attacks or *angina,* chest pain caused by narrowing of the coronary arteries. Studies indicate that beta-blockers lower the rate of heart attacks. They are most effective in people who are young, white, and have high renin output.

Some of the beta-blockers are somewhat selective, affecting the heart more than the lungs and blood vessels. This is due to the fact that the body actually has two types of beta receptors: the heart has β_1 receptors; the lungs, bronchi, and blood vessels have β_2 receptors. Because of their effect on the lungs, in some people beta-blockers have a tendency to aggravate asthma, emphysema, and bronchitis. They are used with caution in people who have these conditions, or even a history of childhood asthma. Beta-blockers may be contraindicated for people with congestive heart failure, since their cardiac output is already low.

In some people, beta-blockers can cause a variety of central nervous system effects, including depression, vivid dreams, insomnia, and even hallucinations. They can also make an existing depression worse. Because they lower cardiac output, beta-blockers sometimes cause leg cramps, as well as cold hands and feet in low temperatures. Such side effects vary with the individual and the particular drug, and they often disappear if the drug is switched. Like diuretics, beta-blockers cause a rise in cholesterol level and can cause impotence in men. The latter problem can be alleviated by decreasing the dosage or by switching drugs. Beta-blockers can also cause fatigue and/or lethargy, and a lowered tolerance for heavy exercise. For this reason, they are not recommended for people who do very rigorous exercise programs.

Angiotensin-converting enzyme (ACE) inhibitors

The *angiotensin-converting enzyme (ACE) inhibitors* are a group of drugs that lower blood pressure by preventing the renin-angiotensin system from contracting the muscle fibers in the walls of the arterioles. Renin is an enzyme that is normally produced by the kidneys in response to a drop in blood pressure. In some people with hypertension, renin is constantly produced in greater than normal amounts. Upon entering the bloodstream, renin breaks down a specific protein, producing angiotensin I. When angiotensin I passes through the lungs, it encounters angiotensin-converting enzyme (ACE), which is present in the lungs in high amounts. ACE converts angiotensin I to angiotensin II, a powerful vasoconstrictor that causes immediate constriction of the arterioles, thereby directly raising blood pressure. ACE inhibitors stop this cycle, preventing the high amounts of renin from keeping the blood pressure abnormally elevated. ACE inhibitors also reduce sympathetic nervous system activity and stimulate vasodilation.

ACE inhibitors work best in people who are young, white, and have high renin levels, but they are effective for a broad range of people with hypertension. One of their major advantages is that they have far fewer side effects than diuretics or beta-blockers. In fact, most people experience no side effects with ACE inhibitors. In a few people they produce a dry cough, skin rashes, or alterations in the taste of food. ACE inhibitors cause retention of potassium and excretion of sodium, both of which are valuable for people with hypertension. Because of these effects, people on ACE inhibitors generally should not take potassium supplements, nor should they be on a severely salt restricted diet. ACE inhibitors are very powerful in combination with diuretics. Another important advantage of ACE inhibitors is that they do not affect cholesterol levels, which makes them very good for people with high cholesterol levels or other risk factors for heart disease. Unlike some of the other types of drugs, ACE inhibitors do not produce fatigue, exercise intolerance, sexual dysfunction, or depression.

Calcium channel blockers

Calcium channel blockers, or *calcium antagonists,* are another new class of antihypertensives that are frequently prescribed because of their effectiveness and relative lack of side effects. Calcium is necessary for contraction of the smooth muscles that line the walls of the small arteries, and it affects the *pacemaker,* the area of the heart which determines how fast the heart beats. Calcium channel blockers inhibit the transport of calcium into the muscle cells of the heart and small arteries by actually blocking the channel through which calcium enters the cell. As a result, the muscle cells are relaxed and the small arteries dilate, causing a decrease in peripheral resistance and a drop in blood pressure. Some calcium channel blockers slow the heart rate slightly, others do not. Calcium channel blockers are effective in a broad range of people with hypertension, but are most often recommended for people with low renin levels. They are more likely to be effective in blacks and older people than either ACE inhibitors or beta-blockers. Because of their effect on the heart, calcium channel blockers are very effective for people who have angina or certain arrhythmias as well as hypertension.

Side effects vary with the three different types of calcium channel blockers, but are uncommon. Dizziness and/or lightheadedness, and swelling of the ankles can occur temporarily when the drug is first started, but usually disappear with time. Headache or constipation can occur with some calcium channel blockers. Calcium channel blockers may be contraindicated in people with certain heart conditions.

Other antihypertensive drugs

There are several other classes of antihypertensive drugs that are not generally used for initial therapy, but are given in combination with other drugs when blood pressure reduction is not totally successful with initial medications. These drugs may have more frequent side effects, especially in higher doses, but they provide doctors with even greater flexibility in the treatment of hypertension. The first three types are sympathetic nervous system inhibitors, the fourth are vasodilators.

The first group, *centrally acting adrenergic inhibitors* (also known as *centrally acting alpha-blockers* or *antagonists*), work on the central nervous system. They directly stimulate α_2 receptors in the brain stem, which stops the flow of impulses to the sympathetic nervous system, thereby causing blood vessel dilation which drops blood pressure. These drugs are often used in conjunction with diuretics or ACE inhibitors because they can cause salt and water retention. Some of the centrally acting adrenergic inhibitors can cause significant side effects, including sedation, fatigue, dryness of the mouth, dizziness upon arising, diarrhea or constipation, and impotence in men. These side effects are generally worst when the drug is started and often disappear over time.

DRUGS USED TO TREAT HIGH BLOOD PRESSURE

Drug(s)	Dosage	Common side effects	Comments
Diuretics			
Hydrochlorothiazide	12.5–100 mg daily	Lowers potassium, calcium, and magnesium; raises cholesterol, uric acid, and glucose. Rash, impotence (in men), fatigue.	Can trigger gout. Increases drug levels of lithium.
Chlorthalidone	12.5–50 mg. daily		
Metolazone	2.5–5.0 mg daily		
Indapamide	2.5–5.0 mg daily		
Beta-adrenergic receptor blocking agents, or beta-blockers			
Acebutolol	400–1200 mg in 1–2 doses daily	Slow heart rate, wheezing, fatigue, cold hands and feet, depression, insomnia, impotence (in men), raised triglyceride levels, lowered HDLs (except for Pindolol and Acebutolol).	Avoided in people with asthma, heart failure, some arrhythmias, diabetes, and peripheral vascular disease.
Atenolol	50–200 mg daily		
Metoprolol	50–200 mg in 1–2 doses daily		
Nadolol	20–160 mg daily		
Pindolol	5–20 mg twice daily		
Propranolol	20–160 mg twice daily		
Timolol	5–10 mg twice daily		
Angiotensin-converting enzyme (ACE) inhibitors			
Captopril	50–300 mg in 2–3 doses daily	Skin rash, taste disturbances, cough.	
Analapril	5–40 mg in 1–2 doses daily		
Lisinopril	10–40 mg daily		
Calcium channel blockers			
Verapamil	240–480 mg in 1–2 doses daily	Constipation, headache, slow heartbeat.	Avoid in patients with congestive heart failure or slow heart rate (heart block). Interacts with digoxin.

Diltiazem	240–360 mg in 2–3 doses daily	Headache, slow heart rate, foot swelling.	
Nifedipine	20–90 mg. in 2–3 doses daily	Headache, foot swelling, rapid heart rate.	

Centrally acting alpha-blockers or antagonists

Clonidine	0.1–3 mg twice daily	Drowsiness, dry mouth, impotence (in men), fatigue.	Interacts with some antidepressants. Should never be stopped suddenly.
Guanabenz	4–16 mg daily		
Methyldopa	250–1,000 mg daily		

Peripheral-acting adrenergic antagonists

Prazosin	1–10 mg twice daily	Dizziness or fainting with first dose, headache, weakness, palpitations.	
Terazosin	1–10 mg in 1–2 doses daily		
Guanethidine	10–100 mg daily	Lightheadedness on standing, diarrhea, impotence (in men).	
Guanadrel	5–20 mg twice daily		
Reserpine	0.1–25 mg. daily	Nasal stuffiness, depression, may aggravate stomach ulcers.	Stop if people become depressed.

Vasodilators

Hydralazine	25–200 mg twice daily	Headache, rapid heart rate.	Stop if chest pain or palpitations occur.
Minoxidil	5–20 mg twice daily	Headache, rapid heartbeat, growth of hair on face and extremities.	

A second class, closely related to the centrally acting adrenergic inhibitors, are called the *peripheral-acting adrenergic inhibitors* (also known as *peripheral-acting adrenergic antagonists*). These drugs block the release of norepinephrine from nerve endings in the blood vessel walls. As a result, the arterioles cannot constrict, so blood pressure drops.

A third class is called *alpha-adrenergic blockers*. They work by blocking the alpha receptors in the blood vessels, causing relaxation in the smooth muscles of the small arteries, and thereby lowering peripheral resistance. They can cause a variety of side effects, including heart palpitations, headache, and nervousness. They also cause a marked drop in blood pressure, which sometimes causes fainting after the first dose. Alpha-adrenergic blockers are generally given in combination with diuretics.

A fourth class, *vasodilators,* work by directly relaxing the muscles in the walls of the small arteries. Vasodilators are not used alone because they can cause a speedup in heartbeat. They are generally given with beta-blockers, which slow down heart rate, and with diuretics. Their most common side effects are headaches, palpitations, and fluid retention (hence their use in combination with diuretics).

Fixed medicine combinations

A number of patients who require drugs to control their hypertension are best managed with a combination of several drugs. Combinations often allow lower dosages to be used, and they have the advantage of approaching the problem through several physiological mechanisms. Since in most cases hypertension is the result of more than one causal factor, combination therapies are likely to be more effective than a single drug. Once the most effective combination is determined, some doctors prescribe fixed-dose combination tablets that contain both drugs in the appropriate amounts. Most of these tablets consist of a diuretic plus one of the other classes of drugs. A fixed-dose tablet simplifies a person's regimen, and is often less expensive. The disadvantage to fixed-dose combinations is that the dosages are less flexible and therefore may not be exactly tailored to an individual's needs.

Drug interactions

Because antihypertensive drugs broadly affect the physiology of a number of the body's organ systems, including the heart, kidneys and sympathetic nervous system, many high blood pressure medications interact with nonhypertensive medications, both prescription and nonprescription. In fact, some combinations of antihypertensive drugs even combine to produce too radical a drop in blood pressure, or create imbalances in potassium levels. Since the doctor determines the dosages and types of antihypertensive drugs, their interaction is generally not a problem, but the doctor may not be aware of other medications a patient takes. Thus it is important that people inform their doctor about any other drugs they take, even occasionally.

Some nonhypertensive drugs block the effectiveness of antihypertensive medications and can result in a person's blood pressure remaining higher than it should be. Aspirin and nonsteroidal anti-inflammatory compounds, both prescription (e.g., *Indocin*) and nonprescription

---

HYPERTENSION DRUG INTERACTIONS

Diuretics
Can raise blood levels of the drug lithium.
Effectiveness can be blocked by nonsteroidal anti-inflammatories.

Beta-blockers
Effectiveness of Propranolol may be reduced by some cholesterol-lowering drugs.
May reduce breakdown of drugs metabolized by the liver (e.g., lidocaine, coumarin, chlorpromazin).

Angiotensin-converting enzyme (ACE) inhibitors
Interact with nonsteroidal anti-inflammatory drugs to cause potassium retention.

Calcium channel blockers
May cause increase in digoxin levels.
May react with quinidine to drop blood pressure below normal levels.

(e.g., *Advil*), antagonize diuretics and ACE inhibitors. People on these antihypertensive drugs should not take aspirin or nonsteroidal anti-inflammatory drugs without consulting their physician.

There are a number of other common drug interactions. Some calcium channel blockers interact with the heart medicine *digoxin,* causing heart rate to slow. Diuretics enhance the absorption of lithium by the kidneys. Some peripheral-acting adrenergic inhibitors are blocked by *ephedrine,* a decongestant, and by some antidepressants. Similarly, some beta-blockers interact with cholesterol-lowering drugs, as well as with calcium channel blockers and some peripheral-acting adrenergic inhibitors. Oral steroids or steroid injections can drop the levels of potassium, and therefore should not be used with drugs that lower potassium, such as diuretics.

Working out a personal treatment program with your doctor

An active patient generally works out the best antihypertensive regimen. Research backs up this assertion. One study on hypertension showed that when doctors addressed patients as partners, informed them of the reason for drug therapy and how the drug worked, encouraged them to report side effects, and worked with them to optimize drug dosages, much better control over blood pressure was achieved. It is really to everyone's advantage if people take an active part in their drug therapy, rather than leave it all up to the doctor.

The first step in becoming an active patient is knowledge. Everyone being treated for hypertension should be aware of what the major kinds of antihypertensive drugs do, and what their common side effects are. It's important that people realize that side effects can be minimized by adjusting dosages or switching drugs. The ideal adjustment of medication can be achieved only when a person understands what's happening, and works with the doctor to achieve the best choice of drugs. If the doctor isn't told about side effects, he or she can't do anything to lessen them. Ask your doctor about side effects and/or read about them (see chart). Remember, not everyone experiences side effects; in fact, most people do not, especially if drug dosages are low.

Pay attention to how you feel, noting whether you experience any side effects, how bothersome they are, and how frequently they occur.

Notify your doctor in detail about any side effects you do notice and discuss how much they bother you. Ask your doctor how the drugs can be adjusted to make you feel better without sacrificing the goal of adequately controlling your blood pressure. Remember that each person's reaction to medication is individual, both in terms of effectiveness and side effects. Making adjustments in medication does not mean the doctor isn't acting knowledgeably or scientifically, rather it reflects sensitivity to the patient's needs. Although the doctor will try to minimize the number of pills and the number of times medication is taken each day, it is useful to have a weekly medication box or chart. To make taking your pills a habit that is easily remembered, it is best to take your medication at fixed times or points in your daily schedule, for example, after meals. The goal of working with the doctor is to jointly evaluate whether medication is working optimally, or adjustments need to be made. Trust your own feelings; if you do not feel well on a drug, it is probably not good for you.

There are several common obstacles to optimizing drug therapy. The most important is attitude. People who see their physician as an authority who knows best, rather than as a partner, are least likely to question their doctor or complain about side effects. Other people have negative attitudes toward drugs, and see themselves as weak because they need drugs, or see drugs as poisons rather than as helpers. People who are dissatisfied with their drug regimen for any reason are likely to stop taking their medication or to take it irregularly. Studies have shown that this is the most significant problem in control of hypertension. Research shows that over half of all patients stop taking medication completely, and another quarter have poor blood pressure control. An active partnership between doctor and patient results in the fewest side effects and the best blood pressure control. Remember, it is you, not the doctor, who takes the medication and derives the benefits.

CHAPTER SEVEN

Hypertension and Sexuality

A satisfactory sex life should be one of the goals of any *take charge* approach to hypertension. Provided a person does not have uncontrolled moderate-to-severe high blood pressure, sex is no more dangerous than any form of exercise that raises heartbeat and blood pressure. Although it is not uncommon for men with hypertension to have problems with sexual dysfunction, such problems can almost always be alleviated. Much of the time these problems are the result of specific high blood pressure medications, and they disappear when the dosage is lowered or another drug is substituted. However, in recent years doctors have begun to recognize that emotional concerns about life and health may also cause men with high blood pressure to have sexual problems. In either case, by working with their doctor, men can usually resolve these problems.

Because a definite percentage of men with high blood pressure complain of sexual problems, a number of studies have been done on hypertension and sexual dysfunction in men, but no corresponding studies have been done on women. Failure for a man to maintain an erection is an obvious impediment to both partners' fulfillment, whereas changes in a woman's arousal are more subtle and may not even be reported to doctors. Interestingly, the research on sexual dysfunction and hypertension shows that the issue is quite complex, and often involves more than a simple side effect of a drug. It is important to realize that prevalence of sexual dysfunction increases with age in any group of men, whether they are hypertensive or not. As early as 1948, Kinsey reported that 2% of men experienced problems with erection at 40 years of age, 7% by age 55, and 25% by age 70. More recent studies have shown the incidence to be even higher. Among 40-year-old, heterosexual men in stable relationships, about 10% experience sexual problems, and this percentage rises with age.

Numerous studies have shown that a greater number of men on antihypertensive medications experience sexual problems than among a comparable group of men who do not have high blood pressure. In fact, impotence is one of the most common reasons for switching medication among men with high blood pressure. In different drug studies, men on specific diuretics show between a 3% and a 32% incidence of impotence. With various beta-blockers, impotence rates vary between 7% and 23%. Again, it must be emphasized that the problem is not simply the result of a given drug, since the great majority of men taking any of the drugs do not experience sexual dysfunction. The problem lies in the particular *combination* of an individual, a specific drug, and the dosage.

Further research has complicated this seemingly clear drug-dosage-individual theory. Several studies have shown that men with *untreated* hypertension have a slightly higher rate of sexual dysfunction than a comparable group of men with normal blood pressure. This raises a question as to whether something in the nature of the disease itself may impair sexual function. The problem may be related to sympathetic arousal or blood flow. Or the problem may be emotional in nature. There may even be another explanation that plays a role. In one study, a group of men who actually had normal blood pressure were led to believe that they had mild hypertension. Although they were not given any medication whatsoever, this group experienced twice the incidence of impotence normally seen in men their age, which in fact corresponds to the level of sexual problems seen in men with mild hypertension which has not been treated with drugs. These results have led researchers to speculate that telling men they are hypertensive may affect their sexual function. This response is referred to as the "labeling effect."

Giving people a reason to think of themselves as "sick" may have far-reaching effects in terms of their outlook and sexual function.

Other research raises even more questions. One study found that hypertensive men showed the same rates of impotence regardless of whether they were treated with an antihypertensive medication or with a *placebo,* a tablet containing no active substance. These results substantiate the idea that people are emotionally affected by the feeling that they're "ill," or by the belief that a drug may have side effects. Finally, some research seems to indicate that among hypertensive men, those who receive medication and those who do not have equally elevated rates of impotence. This would also indicate that factors other than drugs may play an important role in their sexual dysfunction.

The physiology of the male sexual response

Everyone knows that sexual response varies with mood, environment, changes in physiology, health, day-to-day problems, etc. Physiologists have done a great deal of research on the physiology of normal sexual functioning among males. They conclude that sexual arousal is the result of several factors: input from all the sense organs (eyes, ears, nose, taste buds), mental images or fantasies, and tactile stimulation in the genital region. Sights, sounds, odors, and tastes combine with fantasy to stimulate the cerebral cortex of the brain, which sends out impulses via the sympathetic branch of the autonomic nervous system. At the same time, tactile stimulation of the penis is registered in the spinal cord, which stimulates the parasympathetic branch of the autonomic nervous system. Within the penis, the autonomic nervous system controls the opening of muscle sphincters in the artery walls and the closing of sphincters in the walls of the veins. Dilation of arterial sphincters allows more blood to enter the cavernous spaces in the arterial network within the penis, while the closing of venous sphincters prevents the blood from returning to the body as it normally does. These mechanisms cause the penis to become erect by filling with four to eleven times the normal amount of blood. Interestingly, the pressure needed within the arteries of the penis to create an erection is only 85–105 mmHg. Both the hormone *testosterone* and the hormone *prolactin* (which causes milk production in females), as well as many neurotransmitters, play a role in making the penis erect. For men to experience erections, the three mechanisms—the autonomic nervous system and associated neurotransmitters, the hormonal system, and blood flow—have to work correctly and harmoniously. If any of these systems are sufficiently disturbed, a man may have problems with sexual dysfunction. As we discussed in the chapter on drugs, some types of antihypertensive drugs work by affecting the sympathetic nervous system, others affect blood flow or blood volume, and a few even affect hormone production.

Like other forms of physical exertion, intercourse raises blood pressure. In a study of nonhypertensive men it was found that, at rest, the average blood pressure was 112/66 with a pulse of 67. Among this same group, blood pressure was 148/79 with a pulse of 136 upon insertion of the penis into the vagina, and was 163/81 with a pulse of 189 at the point of orgasm. These values are very similar to those of people who are engaging in aerobic exercise. Just as exercise is not dangerous for people whose hypertension is under control, neither is sex. On the other hand, just as strenuous exercise can be dangerous for people with *untreated* moderate-to-severe hypertension, sex can be too since it raises blood pressure by an average of 50 points systolic and 15 points diastolic. Normally, this is not dangerous, but it can be if people's blood pressure is very high to begin with. If a person's average blood pressure is higher than 175/110, he (or she) should consult the doctor about having sexual intercourse. Many doctors recommend refraining from sex, as well as vigorous exercise, until blood pressures above this value can be brought under better control.

How specific antihypertensive drugs affect sexual function

Because many antihypertensive drugs affect blood flow and/or sympathetic nervous system activity, they can cause problems with sexual function in some individuals. But it is important to reiterate that most individuals on these medications do not have problems, and that factors other than high blood pressure or antihypertensive drugs can cause sexual problems in men over 40.

As a group, *diuretics* have been found to impair sexual function in a definite percentage of the men who take them. The percentage varies widely in different studies, from 3% to 32%. The most commonly used diuretics are the *thiazides*. It is not known specifically how they affect sexual functioning, but presumably they simply lower blood flow to the penis. Another type of diuretic, *spironolactone,* which is a potassium-sparing diuretic, actually suppresses production of the male sex hormone *androgen.* Doctors have also found that combining diuretics with other antihypertensive drugs causes a higher incidence of impotence than using diuretics alone.

The *beta-blockers* lower heartbeat and cardiac output by blocking receptor sites on the heart muscle that pick up neurotransmitters from the sympathetic nervous system. It is not clear how beta-blockers contribute to impotence, but they may affect sympathetic arousal generally, and they do limit the amount of blood being pumped by the heart during exercise. Studies show that the number of men experiencing sexual problems with this type of drug rose sharply as dosage went up, and also increased when beta-blockers were used in combination with other drugs.

Two types of antihypertensive drugs which affect the sympathetic nervous system are less commonly used. They are the *centrally acting* and the *peripheral-acting adrenergic inhibitors.* Both affect sexual function by altering the sympathetic nervous system's ability to control blood vessel dilation and contraction. Within these two categories, some medications affect sexual performance in a high number of men, others in a low number.

The newer drugs, *ACE inhibitors* and *calcium channel blockers* have far fewer side effects than either diuretics or beta-blockers. In particular, they have not been associated with impotence problems in many men. For this reason, they are increasingly prescribed.

General advice on sexuality and hypertension

By making lifestyle changes and working with the doctor, virtually everyone can successfully control their blood pressure and continue to enjoy a satisfactory sex life. Because there is some association between sexual dysfunction and a number of antihypertensive medications, it is preferable whenever possible to control blood pressure with lifestyle modifications. The major lifestyle changes include diet, exercise, and stress reduction. Losing weight, getting in shape, dealing with emotional issues, and/or learning to relax more effectively will not only help to lower blood pressure, they will also have a positive effect on a person's sex life. Relaxation and dealing with emotional issues are particularly important because anxiety and depression are linked to many problems with sexual function.

If satisfactory control cannot be achieved without drugs, lifestyle changes should not simply be abandoned. Not only do the positive effects of lifestyle alterations remain important, they can often lower blood pressure enough to allow a reduction in the dosage of medication people take. The lower the dosage of any antihypertensive medication, the less likely it will contribute to problems with sexual functioning.

Many things can help to lessen the likelihood of experiencing sexual problems as a result of antihypertensive medication. First of all, it is important to acknowledge that sexual dysfunction is an emotional topic for most men. For many middle-aged men the inability to maintain an erection is a new, and perhaps embarrassing, problem. Like women in this age group, men may find they have a longer response time. Becoming anxious about it only compounds the problem. Acceptance of changes in lovemaking patterns and open communication with one's partner is particularly important and is most likely to elicit support.

Equally important is frank, open communication with the doctor. In particular, the doctor should be aware of whether or not people have had any sexual problems *before* going on medication, and what the nature of those problems was. Ongoing, unresolved problems are likely to continue, and should not be attributed to medication. There are a number of physical and psychological causes for sexual dysfunction which can be diagnosed and dealt with independently from hypertension. In the course of working out an effective program for blood pressure control, questions about sexual function commonly come up in evaluating antihypertensive medications. Thus it is a natural time to deal with sexual problems.

With the number of drugs presently available, the doctor has a great deal of leeway in the specific drug and dosage that are prescribed. If people start on a drug and experience sexual problems, they should promptly communicate these problems to their doctor, who will do one of three things: stop the drug, lower the dosage, or switch to another medication. One of these strategies is almost always effective if the problem is drug related.

When starting any hypertensive medication it is important that people go into the situation with an open mind—even a positive attitude—and assume they *won't* have problems with the drug, not that they *will*. As we mentioned earlier, a number of people with hypertension develop problems with sexual function even when they are put on a placebo (an inactive drug). Presumably this is the result of worrying about their health, or becoming anxious about the idea that medication may have adverse effects. A positive attitude will help to alleviate these concerns and will help to deal with sexual problems if they do arise.

Taking charge of your hypertension includes dealing with your sexuality. Close communication with your doctor will help you to arrive at the most effective treatment program, including lifestyle changes as well as drugs. Like the rest of the *take charge* program, dealing with hypertension and sexuality involves setting positive goals, taking action, and working with your doctor. In this case, the goal is to enjoy a satisfactory sex life without sacrificing good blood pressure control. It should not be a choice between one or the other. By resolving sexual problems *and* maintaining good blood pressure control, people can enjoy physical satisfaction as well as long-term good health.

CHAPTER EIGHT

Staying in Charge

This final chapter of the book is about putting together all the elements in the *take charge* program in order to achieve long-term maintenance of normal blood pressure. To do this, you will need an ongoing evaluation of the program you have developed. How successful is the program? Which aspects are effective, which are not? Think over each of the areas to see which ones you are enjoying, and which are troublesome. As you gain more knowledge about and experience with hypertension, consider what other approaches you would like to try. Would more stress reduction be helpful? Are you more interested in diet than you were at first? Honestly evaluate the changes you have not been very successful at making. Do you find you are still eating more salt than you should? Consider why you are having trouble with those things that are problematic, and how you can improve the situation.

Taking charge of your health

As we've said, the *take charge* program is divided into four steps. The first step is the *decision to take charge* of your hypertension. This step is based on a clear understanding of the fact that high blood pressure can result in serious illness if it is allowed to go untreated. Hopefully, this knowledge will motivate you to set a realistic goal for lowering your blood pressure. The same information that motivated you to take charge should motivate you to achieve long-range blood pressure control. Maintaining motivation is the key to successful, long-term treatment.

The second step, *taking action*, involves the development of lifestyle changes and/or a drug program. This step depends upon knowledge of how lifestyle factors and drugs lower blood pressure. When people learn that a particular intervention has been shown to be effective, they are motivated to try it. This step also involves gaining greater knowledge of yourself, and developing good communication with your doctor. This chapter deals with the third and fourth steps, *taking control of your treatment* and *maintaining optimum treatment over time*.

Taking control of your treatment

Taking control of your treatment involves monitoring your blood pressure at regular intervals in the doctor's office, and perhaps at home. Only by keeping track of your blood pressure can the effectiveness of treatment be evaluated. Based on your blood pressure response and on how you feel, you can work with your doctor to make adjustments in your lifestyle and/or your medications. Only you know how well you are complying with suggested lifestyle changes, and only you can evaluate how the drugs make you feel.

Home monitoring is not just a matter of taking your blood pressure. It is important for people to realize that their blood pressure goes up and down in response to a number of factors. It has been mentioned that blood pressure tends to go up during the day, when people exercise, and, of course, when they feel under stress. Occasional high values, within a range set by the doctor, are normal and do not mean treatment is not effective. People should take their blood pressure at a fixed time of day after having rested for 5–10 minutes—not just when they feel stressed or anxious that it is high. What is important to the doctor is your average resting value, not just your blood pressure when you are under maximum stress. If people become alarmed each time they take their blood pressure at home, and it causes them to worry even more, it may be counterproductive to do home monitoring. In this situation home monitoring simply serves to make people more upset, and the values they record may not be true resting values. It is also worthwhile for people to take their blood pressure cuff in to their doctor's office to see that it is properly calibrated and that they are using it correctly. Sometimes electronic cuffs or inexpensive devices are not very accurate, and in this case incorrect figures may be worse than no figures at all. The value of home monitoring is to demonstrate the success of your program. It's like weighing yourself to see if a diet is working. Successful lowering of blood pressure shows that the regimen you have undertaken is working.

Maintaining your program and working with your doctor

The fourth step, *maintaining optimum treatment over time,* is based on developing and maintaining healthy lifestyle habits and working with the doctor. Crucial to long-term control is a change in your own attitudes, and the support of family and friends. Cooperation and communication with the doctor is important because, over time, changes in blood pressure can occur and side effects from medication can develop. Also, new and improved drugs are becoming available all the time. Once a satisfactory program is established, it should be evaluated with the doctor on a regular basis. Drug dosages may need to be adjusted to minimize side effects, or new drugs may be substituted. If lifestyle changes are very effective, a step-down alternative may be tried in which drugs are decreased or even eliminated.

In terms of the lifestyle part of the program, it is important to realize that the work is ongoing. Dealing with stress truly involves the core of one's personality and outlook on the world. Habitual patterns of arousal are generally deeply ingrained by adulthood and are often slow to change. For anyone, a path of personal growth and spiritual fulfillment is a lifelong task. A long-term program for taking charge of your blood pressure merges with lifelong goals for happiness and fulfillment.

All of the lifestyle changes that contribute to lowering your blood pressure will contribute to your health and happiness in broader and deeper ways. The stress reduction part of the program will give you better control over your own emotional states, and the ability to deal with troublesome situations more effectively. As you get better at stress reduction, not only is your blood pressure likely to drop, your life will improve. The dietary changes that are recommended for hypertension take into account mankind's evolutionary roots, and thus are broadly beneficial in preventing a number of diseases. Healthier nutrition will also help to make you look and feel better. Likewise, the exercise part of the program will have physical and psychological benefits that go far beyond controlling high blood pressure. Not only will regular exercise make you look and feel better, it will improve your mental outlook. Even the drug part of the program can give you skills in paying attention to your body, communicating your feelings to others, making your needs known, and working for positive change.

From a program such as this, you learn to participate actively in your own health care. As an adjunct, you may find yourself learning to become more active in other areas of your life, and better able to deal with situations you cannot completely control. Changing attitudes and habits are processes that are deep-seated and ongoing. A few European studies suggest that significant psychological growth, followed by a change in arousal patterns, may be able to reverse the physiology of disease, and even cure hypertension.

Blood pressure and self-confidence

Almost all studies on hypertension have shown that for many people improvement takes place *without* treatment in the year after their condition is first diagnosed. This phenomenon, which is most common in people with mild hypertension, is referred to as the "placebo effect." It was discovered when a significant percentage of the control group in most randomized studies, to whom "nothing" was done, showed a drop in blood pressure. The drop was so significant that no hypertension studies are done now without a control group because researchers recognize that a positive change may be due to the placebo effect rather than to whatever intervention is being studied. The question is, why did people's blood pressure go down in the control groups? Obviously, "no treatment" actually represented some kind of treatment. In fact, the people in the control groups were diagnosed, followed by a doctor, told that they were being treated (and perhaps even given a pharmacologically nonactive pill), and that they were expected to get better (since the doctor didn't know which people were in the treatment group as opposed to the control group).

In trying to explain these unexpected placebo results, researchers theorize that those people in the control group whose blood pressure dropped understood they had an illness, thought they were being treated, and believed that they would get better. In fact, no medical treatment was actually given, except for reassurance. Clearly, the people got better by themselves, either because of a change in psychological outlook, or possibly because of self-imposed lifestyle changes. Studies such as these underscore how important it is for people to take charge of their own health. The control groups in these studies were successfully able to lower their blood pressure for reasons that are not completely understood. Although the explanations for this phenomenon are unproven, the blood pressure drop they experienced was real.

Other studies have also demonstrated significant blood pressure decreases due to unexplained factors. Several things were common to all these studies: the people were aware that their blood pressure was high and wanted to lower it, and most likely they had some belief in their treatment. One study dealt with relaxation, biofeedback or imagery as interventions. Compared to a control group, the group who used these techniques achieved greater reductions in blood pressure. The greatest decrease was obtained with a combination of relaxation and imagery. Interestingly, the researchers found that a drop in blood pressure occurred whether or not people's muscles actually relaxed, or they did the exercises regularly. The results were certainly puzzling, and the researchers could only conclude that stress reduction techniques did work, but the mechanisms by which they worked were unclear.

In a study dealing with diet, it was found that there was a minimum drop in blood pressure when people changed only one nutritional factor, such as sodium, potassium, calcium, fat, or fiber. But when people changed all these factors, a significant drop in blood pressure occurred. This may simply be because the factors are additive, or because the response of blood pressure is both more complex and more "global."

Learning to lower blood pressure

Barry Dworkin, a researcher at Penn State, has developed a broad theory of hypertension that is unproven but thought-provoking. Dworkin believes that high blood pressure is a learned response that certain people develop as a means of dealing with unpleasant situations. The mechanisms that Dworkin postulates are intriguing. He points out that pressure receptors in the carotid arteries of the neck are stimulated when blood pressure rises. In both humans and animals, stimulating these receptors causes relaxation and even pleasure, and lowers the response to aversive stimuli such as noise or stress. Dworkin theorizes that in susceptible people or animals a blood pressure rise during sympathetic arousal stimulated the pressure receptors and lessened the anxiety they felt. Dworkin believes that people eventually learn to raise their blood pressure in order to lower the anxiety they feel. Such a response could have resulted from the body integrating a pleasure response with the fight-or-flight response. In that way, people who were constantly under stress would benefit from it. Ultimately, they may even become addicted to the norepinephrine "rush" that accompanies anxiety and tension. Dworkin theorizes that in some people who have high blood pressure, the body is actually attempting to maintain constant high levels of stress hormones.

We believe that if people have learned such a response, it is possible for them to unlearn it. To accomplish this, they have to be able to distinguish between feelings of arousal and feelings of relaxation, and then "learn" how to relax, especially after arousal. Moreover, they have to learn to get pleasure from the relaxed state, as well as from the aroused state. Many people in our culture believe that the aroused state is the productive state, the one in which things get done. They have forgotten how to accomplish tasks in a steady, relaxed manner. It is important for people to learn that pleasure can come from inside, and that they can experience pleasure without raising their blood pressure. If they can change their attitude or world view, they can ultimately change how they react to aversive stimuli.

We mention these three provocative studies in order to encourage people to think more broadly about the whole subject of hypertension. It is our belief that taking charge of your blood pressure is a global process that involves both mind and body. Although the exact mechanisms are unknown, making lifestyle changes and participating actively in your drug therapy have both been proven to lower blood pressure. At a more general level, taking charge involves relearning our ways of reacting to the world. It involves learning to take pleasure in small things and actively changing our ability to handle stressful situations. It involves improving our capacity to control our need for immediate gratification, whether it be in eating or in accomplishing tasks. It involves our ability to pay attention to our bodies and to communicate our needs to others.

We invite you to make lowering your blood pressure part of enriching your life and feeling healthier. We believe that by working actively with your doctor to take charge of your hypertension, you can do this.

Bibliography

Chapter 1: Taking Charge

Patient Behavior for Blood Pressure Control. Guidelines for Professionals. 1979. *Journal of the American Medical Association* 241:2534.

Reiter, J. 1987. *Taking Control of Your Epilepsy*. The Basics.

Schulman, B. 1979. "Active Patient Orientation and Outcomes in Hypertensive Treatment." *Medical Care* 17:267.

Chapter 2: What Is Hypertension?

The Joint National Committee. 1988. "The 1988 Report of the Joint National Committee on Detection, Evaluation, and Treatment of High Blood Pressure." *Archives of Internal Medicine* 148:1023.

Braunwald, E. 1984. *Heart Disease: A Textbook of Cardiovascular Medicine*. W. B. Saunders.

Hypertension Detection and Follow-Up Program. 1979. "Five-Year Findings of the Hypertension Detection and Follow-Up Program." *Journal of the American Medical Association* 242:2562.

Kaplan, N. 1990. "The Potential Benefits of Non-Pharmacological Therapy." *The American Journal of Hypertension* 3:425.

McCanon, D. 1984. "Diuretic Therapy for Mild Hypertension: The Real Cost of Treatment." *American Journal of Cardiology* 53:9A.

Krup, M. 1988. *Current Medical Diagnosis and Treatment*. Appleton and Lang.

Laragh, J. H. 1990. *Hypertension: Pathophysiology, Diagnosis, and Management*. Raven Press.

Petersdorf, R. 1991. *Harrison's Principles of Internal Medicine*. McGraw-Hill.

Wyngaarden, J. B. 1988. *Cecil Textbook of Medicine*, 18th Edition. W. B. Saunders.

Chapter 3: Hypertension and the Mind

Achterberg, J. 1985. *Imagery and Healing: Shamanism and Modern Medicine*. Shambala.

Antonovsky, A. 1984. "A Sense of Coherence As A Determinant of Health," in Matarazzo, J. *Behavioral Health*. John Wiley & Sons.

Bandura, A. 1977. "Self-Efficacy." *Psychological Review* 84:191–215.

Bandura, A. 1985. "Catecholamine Secretion As A Function of Perceived Coping Self-Efficacy." *Journal of Consulting and Clinical Psychology* 53:3, pp. 406–414.

Beamish, R. E. 1985. *International Symposium on Stress and Heart Disease*, Kluwer Academic Publishers.

Benson, H. 1976. *The Relaxation Response*. Avon Books.

Berkman, L. 1979. "Social Networks, Host Resistance, and Mortality: A 9-Year Follow-Up Study of the Alameda County Residents." *American Journal of Epidemiology* 109:186–204.

Cohen, S. 1986. *Behavior, Health, and Environmental Stress*. Plenum.

Cohen, S. 1985. *Social Support and Health*. Academic Press.

Elliot, R. S. 1984. *Is It Worth Dying For?* Bantam.

Folkow, B. 1958. "Adaptive Structural Changes of the Vascular Wall in Hypertension and Their Relationship to Control of Peripheral Resistance." *Acta Physiology Scandanavia* 44:255.

Goldstein, J. 1983. *The Experience of Insight: A Simple and Direct Guide to Buddhist Meditation*. Shambala Publications.

Henry, J. P. 1977. *Stress, Health, and the Social Environment*. Springer-Verlag.

Holmes, T. H. 1967. "The Social Readjustment Rating Scale." *Journal of Psychosomatic Research* 1:213–218.

Kaplan, M. 1986. "Social Support and Health." *Medical Care* 15:47.

Jacobson, E. 1962. *You Must Relax*. McGraw-Hill.

Kobasa, S. 1983. "Effectiveness of Hardiness, Exercise, and Social Support As Resources Against Illness." *Journal of Psychosomatic Research* 29:525–533.

Muktananda, S. 1980. *Meditate*. State University of New York.

Nuckolls, K. 1972. "Psychological Assets, Life Crises, and the Prognosis of Pregnancy." *American Journal of Epidemiology* 95:431–441.

Ornstein, R. 1987. *The Healing Brain*. Simon & Schuster.

Patel, C. 1985. "Trials of Relaxation in Reducing Coronary Risk." *British Medical Journal of Clinical Research* 290:1103.

Pelletier, K. 1977. *Mind as Healer, Mind as Slayer*. Dell.

Rossman, M. 1987. *Healing Yourself: A Step-By-Step Program for Better Health Through Imagery*. Walker.

Samuels, M. and N. 1975. *Seeing With the Mind's Eye*. Random House.

Schnall, P. L. 1990. "The Relationship Between Job Strain, Workplace Diastolic

Blood Pressure, and Left Ventricular Mass Index." *Journal of the American Medical Association* 263:1929.

Selye, H. 1956. *The Stress of Life*. McGraw-Hill.

Seligman, M. 1975. *Learned Helplessness*. W. H. Freeman.

Shepherd, J. T. 1987. "Conference on Behavioral Medicine and Cardiovascular Disease." *Circulation Monograph* #6, 76 (Supp. I).

Weiss, S. 1986. *Perspectives In Behavioral Medicine*. Academic Press.

Wood, C. 1987. "Are Happy People Healthier?" *Journal of the Royal Society of Medicine* 80:354–356.

Chapter 4: Hypertension and Diet

American Heart Association Committee. 1982. "Rationale for the Diet-Heart Statement of the American Heart Association." *Circulation* 65:839A-851A.

Berglund, A. 1989. "Antihypertensive Effect of Diet Compared with Drug Treatment in Obese Men with Mild Hypertension." *British Medical Journal* 299:480.

Dawber, T. R. 1980. *The Framingham Study*. Harvard University Press.

Eaton, B. 1985. "Paleolithic Genes and 20th Century Health." *Anthroquest* 33:1.

Grumm, R. 1986. "Lipids and Hypertension." *American Journal of Medicine* 80 (Supplement 2A).

Levy, R. I. 1986. "Cholesterol and Coronary Artery Disease." *Journal of the American Medical Association* 80, suppl. 2A, p. 18.

MacMahon, S. W. 1986. "Alcohol and Hypertension." *Annals of Internal Medicine* 105:124.

National Academy of Science/National Research Council Food and Nutrition Board. 1980. *Recommended Dietary Allowances,* 9th Edition. NAS/NRC.

Senate Select Committee on Nutrition and Human Needs. 1977. *Dietary Goals for the U.S.* U.S. Government Printing Office.

Stamler, R. 1989. "Primary Prevention of Hypertension by Nutritional-Hygienic Means." *Journal of the American Medical Association* 262:1801.

U.S. Department of Health, Education, & Welfare. 1979. *Healthy People*. DHEW Publication.

U.S. Department of Health, Education, & Welfare, 1986. *1990 Health Goals for the Nation*. DHEW.

Chapter 5: Hypertension and Exercise

Boger, J. L. 1970. "Exercise, Therapy, and Hypertensive Men." *Journal of the American Medical Association* 211:1668.

Cassel, J. 1971. "Occupation, Physical Activity, and Coronary Heart Disease." *Archives of Internal Medicine* 128:920.

Cooper, K. H. 1976. "Physical Fitness Levels Versus Selected Coronary Risk Factors." *Journal of the American Medical Association* 236:166.

Eaton, B. 1985. "Paleolithic Genes and 20th Century Health." *Anthroquest* 33:1.

Morris, J. N. 1980. "Vigorous Exercise in Leisure-Time: Protection Against Coronary Heart Disease." *Lancet* 8206:1207–1210.

Paffenberger, R. S. 1983. "Physical Activity and the Incidence of Hypertension in College Alumni." *American Journal of Epidemiology* 117:245–256.

Powell, K. E. 1985. "Workshop on Epidemiological and Public Health Aspects of Physical Activity and Exercise: A Summary." *Public Health Reports* 100:118.

Siscoveck, D. S. 1985. "The Disease-Specific Benefits and Risks of Physical Activity and Exercise." Public Health Reports 100:180.

Taylor, T. B. 1985. "The Relationship of Physical Activity and Exercise to Mental Health." *Public Health Reports* 100:195.

Chapter 6: Hypertension Drugs

Laragh, J. H. 1990. *Hypertension: Pathophysiology, Diagnosis, and Management.* Raven Press.

Wyngaarden, J. B. 1988. *Cecil Textbook of Medicine,* 18th Edition. W. B. Saunders.

Chapter 7: Hypertension and Sexuality

Bansal, S. 1988. "Sexual Dysfunction in Hypertensive Men." *Hypertension* 12:1.

Chapter 8: Staying in Charge

Dembroski, T. 1983. *Biobehavioral Bases of Coronary Heart Disease,* Karger.

Meltzer, J. I. 1990. "Physician-Patient Interaction in the Treatment of Hypertension," in Laragh, J. H. *Hypertension.*

Index

141

About the Authors

Mike and Nancy Samuels are committed to teaching people how to take charge of their own health, and they are among the strongest advocates in the medical establishment for preventive medicine and self-care. Mike Samuels, M.D., attended Brown University and graduated from the New York University College of Medicine. Nancy Harrison Samuels is a graduate of Brown University and the Bank Street College of Education. They are the authors of a number of self-help books including *Seeing With the Mind's Eye, The Well Pregnancy Book, The Well Baby Book,* and *The Well Adult.* Mike is also the author of *Healing With the Mind's Eye* and is currently Director of the Art As A Healing Force project, an organization devoted to exploring the connections between art and healing.